Taking Precautions

an intimate history of birth control

Shyama Perera

NEW
HOLLAND

First published in 2004 by New Holland Publishers (UK) Ltd
London · Cape Town · Sydney · Auckland

www.newhollandpublishers.com

Garfield House, 86–88 Edgware Road, London W2 2EA, United Kingdom

80 McKenzie Street, Cape Town 8001, South Africa

14 Aquatic Drive, Frenchs Forest, NSW 2086, Australia

218 Lake Road, Northcote, Auckland, New Zealand

10 9 8 7 6 5 4 3 2 1

ISBN 1 84330 737 5

Publishing Manager: Jo Hemmings
Senior Editor: Kate Michell
Editor: Deborah Taylor
Assistant Editor: Rose Hudson
Indexer: Dorothy Frame
Cover Design and Design: Nicky Barneby
Production: Joan Woodroffe

Reproduction by Pica Digital Pte Ltd, Singapore
Printed and bound in Singapore by Kyodo Printing Co. (Singapore) Pte Ltd

For N and T. Laugh, learn, love and lust, with care.

Taking Precautions

Contents

Introduction

I remember being offered the cap as my first form of contraception. 'Oh, no!', I said, recoiling in horror. 'I don't want to be putting something in there.' The nurse looked at me blankly: 'But that's why you're here isn't it? Because you're putting something in there?'

I was dumbstruck. There is something so deadly serious about birth control, but... it's also utterly humiliating.

Any form of contraception is ultimately concerned with our private parts and the uses thereof. Any questions that are asked in relation to its issue impinge on the most private areas of our lives: our after-dark fantasies and aspirations. No wonder the young and the squeamish balk at discussing such activity with anonymous medical practitioners in white coats.

It takes the romance out of making love; despoils the intimacy of consummation; usurps the role of wanton lust in illicit shagging. Contraception takes the spontaneity out of sex...

Think of it this way: sex is like a Ferrari. It's slick and fast, red and hot, throaty and playful, smooth and seamless. It quickens the pulse and makes you purr: it stirs the loins. But if you don't want to lose your licence, you stick to the speed limit. In other words: acknowledging the need for contraception ruins the fantasy; so, generally, we don't acknowledge it.

And, let's face it, with each new method – gel, sponge, coil, rubbers – there's scope for a 'Carry On' script with Hattie Jacques as Matron, fumbling under the covers as a wide-eyed Barbara Windsor, stirruped and with her legs in the air, squeals: 'Oh dear! Perhaps this wasn't such a good idea...'

The Diversity of Birth-Control Methods

But even without horror or humour, contraception is so diverse, so flexible and so damned *interesting*.

- It has links with the women's suffrage campaign. Running in parallel with the demand that women should have the right to vote was the argument that they should also have the right to regulate their own bodies. The biggest social iniquity of the time was that once women married (particularly if they were at the sharp end of life), their health, well-being and right to self-determination were diminished by serial pregnancies.
- The SAS use condoms as water carriers when living out in the wild. They also use them for storing clean water in countries where the supplies are polluted. This is hardly surprising, as condoms are tested to see if they'll hold the equivalent of nine gallons (forty litres) of air before making it onto the shelf. But blokes who fill condoms with water and pelt each other just for the pure hell of it still come across as missing several brain cells.
- The contents of most contraceptive pessaries from ancient times were food ingredients commonly available on the shelves at the supermarket today. Honey, oil, vinegar, lemon, parsley, thyme, marjoram, sage… And it wasn't a case of old wives' tales – each and every one of these has an effect, depending on how they're administered.
- If you eat a papaya every day, it reduces fertility.
- Vasectomy was once used to stop habitual masturbation. There is a report of a young man with a masturbatory 'problem' visiting an Indiana doctor in 1899 to demand castration to stop his vile and sinful habit (see onanism, page 35). As a compromise, the doctor snipped his tubes instead and the lad stopped his furtive late-night fiddling.
- A Canadian doctor once hoaxed the medical world with a paper on a new contraceptive called Armpitin. He described a series of molecular groups which all bore the chemical make-up 'NO' and

which could be used to hit the olfactory organs. Bizarrely, pharmaceutical companies were taken in and tried to buy the formula.

- More seriously, here are the mortality figures before and after contraception became freely available to both men and women. In Victorian times, one woman died for every 154 live births. By the 1980s, that figure had gone down to the risk being one woman in every 10,000 live births. This isn't just down to contraception releasing women from a disabling cycle of child bearing; antibiotics and improved medical care played their part. In less-developed countries, however, the mortality rates remain shocking; for example, 170 women die per 10,000 live births in Afghanistan.

- And the male pill… It's on its way, but extensive guinea pig trials using cottonseed oil over the last twenty years in China have resulted in many of the guinea pigs becoming permanently sterile.

The Story of Contraception

The facts and figures bedazzle, bewilder and bedevil. There is so much that we don't know that we *should* know. The story of contraception is interwoven with pathos and bathos, humour and humility, ludicrous theorizing and moments of sheer brilliance. And what's interesting is that the movers and shakers haven't always been medical people. For example, the eighteenth-century Italian Lothario Casanova came up with brilliant ideas for stopping sperm from reaching its destiny (see page 61) simply because he needed to devise ways of shooting off into his myriad lovers without facing a paternity suit.

Around the world and across the centuries, the search for reliable birth control has obsessed women and men alike. Tribal people learned the contraceptive properties of plants almost by osmosis. The ancient Greeks noticed the effect of particular vegetation on cattle and successfully tried it out on women. Midwives experimented with emetics and cramp-inducing flora and fauna until they achieved a workable mix. All this happened with very little real information available.

Even now, it is astonishing to think how many of our forebears would have given their stashes of gold to lose their fertility; indeed,

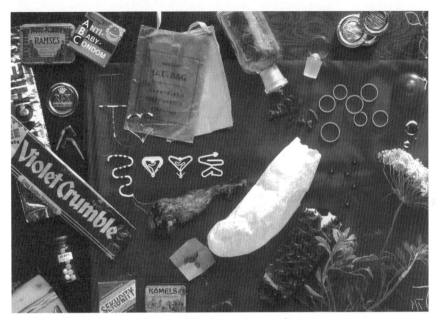

What look like brooches in the middle of this collection of historic contraceptive devices, are in fact forerunners of the IUD or coil. Also here are plants that would have been issued by medieval midwives, sweet wrappers used as substitute condoms by teenagers and variations of the cap.

a number did. One natural contraceptive method recommended by the Greeks – a plant called silphium – had such a huge success rate that its price rose ever higher as stocks shrivelled (see page 25). Ultimately, only the rich could afford it. It is now extinct and we will never know what properties the plant boasted. We can guess that they were significant, however, as the plants were commemorated on the backs of Greek coins.

Silphium's success is a reminder that, while it's the most recent pioneers of birth control who inspire us today, the stalwarts of birth control have always been there – forward-thinking men from as long ago as 1000 BC. It's thanks to them that most women of today can choose with their partners the number of children they want, as well as when in their lives they want to have them.

More recently, Maggie Higgins, who became Margaret Sanger (1883–1966), the American who initiated the search for oral contraception, was driven not by her nursing knowledge, but by the terrible home conditions from whence she came – conditions she blamed for her mother's eleven live births and endless miscarriages, which were followed by an early and miserable death from tuberculosis. Sanger's British counterpart, Marie Stopes (1880–1958), on the other hand, was kicked into touch by an early, sexless marriage that left her frustrated and miserable.

Information, Information, Information

Until the nineteenth century, when it was discovered that women ovulate, the assumption had been that male sperm alone created a baby, and the womb was just the chosen vessel for a developing fetus's containment. Even that view was enlightened compared to that of Stone Age people, who assumed that the Sun and the Moon blessed them with babies.

Yet, there are still people today who are none the wiser. I remember two schoolfriends who got 'caught' in the 1970s – a decade of sexual licence in which the Pill was given out freely, antibiotics were on tap for the slightest infection, and nobody had heard of herpes, HIV or AIDS. The first got pregnant without even knowing she'd made love. It was an encounter at a party with a boy from the same class, and she honestly had no idea that they'd 'done it' behind a curtain in a council flat on the twelfth floor of a central London tower block. Indeed, there was no real evidence of penetration, but heavy petting can be just as dangerous, depending on where a man ejaculates. It was only when my friend's mum noticed she was putting on weight that the accident was discovered. By then, it was too late.

The other friend returned from a Mediterranean holiday to describe, with great humour, a sexual tussle she'd had with a boy on the beach and was mortified to be told by us better-informed young madams, who'd read Molly Parkin's explicit weekly column in the teen-magazine *Petticoat*, that she'd just lost her virginity…

Even in the middle of an information barrage, there are those who just don't know. As one of my acquaintances commented when

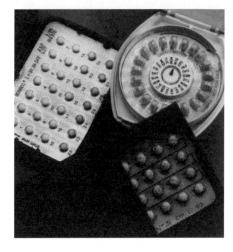

The Pill was originally dispensed in bottles, and later in a rotating pack. Nowadays, it usually comes in a tray form, with each day of the week clearly marked as an aide-mémoire.

I told her I was writing this book: 'Don't times change? When I was younger, you couldn't even discuss sanitary protection with your mother, let alone birth control. Nowadays I go to my friends' houses and their boxes of tampons are on the bathroom window cill for all the world to see and we laugh about flavoured condoms over dinner.'

Morality and Taboos

And that's another reason – the main reason – we should be interested in contraception: to remove the final taboos.

Some of the stories I've come across in researching this book are so bizarre that one wonders where they emanate from. The writings of the Greeks and the practices of larger societies in ancient times are well researched and presented, but other ceremonies and ideas are clearly stitched together from fragments of evidence.

What makes it so difficult to discover the thinking behind some methods, or the exact pattern of them, is that the whole area of fertility, abortion and childbirth has been deliberately shrouded in mystery, both to protect the women who asked for help and those who offered it.

The main reason for such secrecy was the imposition of religious values on entire populations. Before the spread of Christianity, women were able to find recourse to contraception without shame, but after the Church tightened its grip on Europe and the West, only men were offered the opportunity to use protection – and that was more for their sexual health rather than to limit the number of children their wives bore.

Before the arrival of the Pill, only men had access to condoms, and some doctors still demanded the husband's permission before handing out caps and diaphragms to a married woman. This was inevitable in a patriarchal society: babies keep women in their place as homemakers and mothers.

It is a sobering thought to consider that many of the witches burned in medieval times were midwives – women skilled in matters of birth and conception. But contraception is a *woman's right*, because men can't get pregnant. That difference determines the odds of where it is placed on a man's list of priorities and whether or not he takes any responsibility for it.

It is not a coincidence that it was only after the introduction of the Pill and the erosion of taboos that women were able to enter

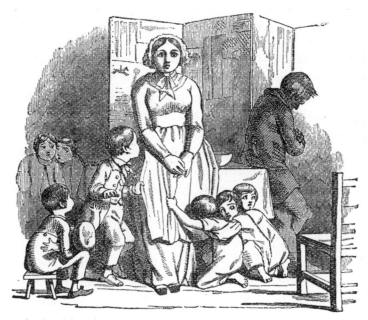

Poor families did not have easy access to what little contraception was available until the 1950s. As a result, in the early twentieth century many women had no choice but to bring up a large family on limited funds.

the job market as equals. It could be argued that the entire sexual revolution was a direct result of the Pill's invention.

The potential gravity of the consequences of unprotected sex for women, however, cannot be emphasized enough. That doesn't mean this book is written specifically for women, because the search for the answer involves and is relevant to both sexes alike. In the pages that follow are large chunks on male contraception, and the future is very much concentrated on finding methods that work for men (see pages 145–57).

But birth control is a *bigger* issue for women, and that is reflected in its history. By pulling back those covers, we open the subject up to everyone in the hope that it helps diminish ignorance and intolerance.

A reporter from a national newspaper once called me and asked: 'Don't you think it's a disgrace that the morning-after pill is available to schoolgirls?' I thought about it for all of a micro-second, weighing up the alternatives. 'I think,' I said, 'that it's less of a problem than schoolgirls having babies and ending up on sink estates unable to finish their education, fulfill their potential as women and be better mothers at a later age.'

Inevitably, morality rears its head when we're discussing contraception, and the world today is very different from the world when those whose names are stamped forever in the firmament of birth control – Aletta Jacobs, Margaret Sanger, Marie Stopes, Katherine McCormick, Margaret Pyke and a whole host more for whom there wasn't space in this book – first started their crusade.

Ironically, they wo-manned the barricades of public sensibility with their bodies covered from head to toe to protect their modesty. They weren't exhorting sexual licence, just liberation from the consequences of sexual pleasure.

Since then, the arguments have changed: contraception is a tool for sexual freedom as well as freedom from pregnancy. In the twenty-first century, we have taken sexual freedom to its ultimate extreme with youngsters stripping off in public and boasting about serial sexual conquests. Whatever one's views on this behaviour, the need is increased to make them aware of the risks. One thing we touch

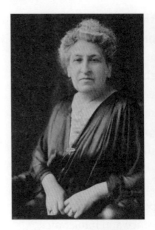
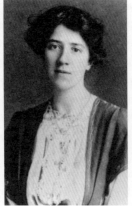
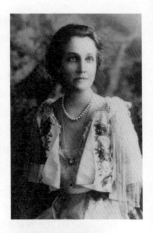
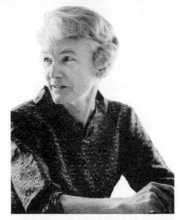
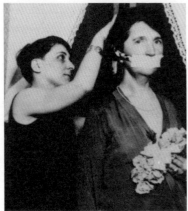

The movers and shakers of the campiagn to liberate women from the impositions of their bodies. Clockwise from top left: Aletta Jacobs (1854–1929), Marie Stopes (1880–1958), Katherine McCormick (1875–1967), Margaret Pyke (1893–1966) Margaret Sanger (1883–1966).

upon in this book is that different forms of contraception suit different lifestyles.

The Issue of Abortion

The single major issue around contraception continues to be abortion (see pages 127–42). Any abortifacient resolution sets the teeth of lobby groups on edge, even if, as is the case with the morning-after pill, it cannot technically displace an egg once fertilized and embedded.

This book does not get involved with the politics of contraception; it merely details the arguments for and against, and documents reasons why ideas may have changed. One example is the physiological change in girls over the centuries, which means that they now menstruate much earlier. Our ancestors could experiment sexually when in their teens and be safe from impregnation. That is not the case for today's youngsters, who have to make adult decisions about their sexuality when they are barely competent enough to keep their keys safe and remember their bus passes.

Inevitably, when we discuss full abortion, the biggest problem is perceived as being that of teenagers using termination as back-up contraception. These are controversial social issues that continue to provoke debate within society and within the health industry.

The Role of the Condom

One thing that hasn't been changed so much as compounded by our physiological, sexual, social and material evolution is the use of the condom as a cover-all solution for the many health issues around sexuality. The condom was first manufactured to prevent the spread of sexual disease (see pages 91–110), and its importance in the field of general good health cannot be overestimated when millions of people are dying from HIV/AIDS.

Figures from the United Nations for the first three years of the twenty-first century put the number of people infected worldwide at 100 million, 45 million of whom are still alive. Half of all sufferers are under the age of twenty-five, many of them children born with the infection. In the United Kingdom, the total figure still remains relatively low, but each year sees a steep increase. This is partly due to the fact that people with AIDS are coming into the United Kingdom from other countries and seeking medical help, however that should not mask the fact that our own base numbers are rising.

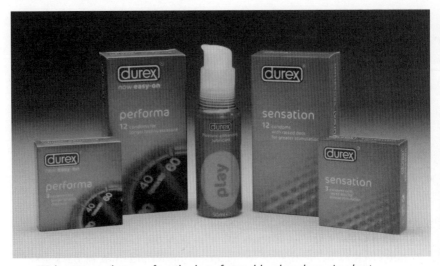

We have come a long way from the days of second-hand condoms, rinsed out and sold to the poor, as a selection from today's Durex range clearly illustrates.

So What is this Book About?

This book will give you some facts and figures about health care, but it does not claim to be a medical aid. Neither does it claim to be an academic study; it is more of a general history. It is an attempt to inform in an entertaining way; to lay bare the theory and experimentation that would lead ultimately to the situation we have today, where contraceptive pills are freely available on the State, and condoms can be bought everywhere: from petrol stations to public toilets to the local shop.

Because, historically, there have always been so many methods of contraception being used disparately across the globe at different times and in different ways, methodologies have been divided up by type (that is, barrier methods, such as the cap, chemical methods, such as the Pill) so there is a sense of how ideas and usage developed in each area of experimentation.

The first two chapters can loosely be described as 'mix-and-match wet' (cervical plugs made from wet ingredients, teas and other medicines) and 'mix-and-match dry' (chastity belts, magic and charms) where odd ideas about birth control that don't necessarily fit any contemporary methods are discussed. From the third chapter onwards, a general timeline begins to emerge, allowing different periods of contraceptive development to be put into context.

Inevitably in a history of contraception, there will be overlaps across the methodologies, but not, I hope, any repetition. The least amount of space is probably given to permanent sterilization because it is not so much a form of birth control, which displaces fertility, as the elective loss of fertility.

This book is also, I hope, a celebration of achievement, and in order to celebrate we must applaud the ridiculous as well as the sublime. It is a pulling together of remedies (from potions to plants) and comedies (stories of cat's livers and weasel's feet) and ideas and ideals, which all play a part in the narrative, if not always with success:

- In Maoist China, women tried swallowing spring tadpoles to ward off conception. Folklore suggested that if a woman drank boiled tadpoles for two days in succession she would become infertile. Interestingly, half the women who took part in a controlled experiment with tadpoles did not fall pregnant. Well, not immediately anyway.
- It is reported that young Moroccan girls who did not want to get pregnant would go into graveyards looking for a fresh grave over which they would step three times in a ritual aimed at preventing pregnancy. The alternative, if they had a dead younger sister, was to go to the sister's grave and shout: 'I don't want any children.'
- Douching has always been popular and there is some sense in the belief that flushing the vagina out after intercourse will help remove sperm. Unfortunately, it's not the slow sperm left behind that make the babies, but those who were first off the mark and are usually well inside the womb before the man's had time to roll off his partner. However, Egyptian women employed douche maids to sluice out their vaginas with a mixture of garlic, wine and

fennel. More recently, women have used Lysol (an antiseptic) and Coca-Cola.

- The American physician Charles Knowlton (1800–1850), who was imprisoned for his writings on birth control (see page 76), came up with a douche of water, salt, vinegar, liquid chloride, zinc sulfite or aluminium potassium sulfite, which was used by nineteenth-century American women for forty years.
- It is reported that French women in medieval times wore the anus and finger of a dead baby round their necks to ward off further babies. The other option, apparently, was popping a milk tooth into an amulet and hanging it from your bottom.
- Britain's leading activist, Marie Stopes (see pages 75–90), was constantly looking for ways of raising money for her clinics. She once wrote to Henry Ford, the man who first made mass-produced cars: 'You are so gloriously rich, and could spare a million or two pounds so easily – won't you send me that right now?'
- Late marriage was favoured in many Western societies as the answer to limiting family size. An aristocratic gentleman would stop having sexual relations with his wife after the birth of an heir – this stopped any future problems of sons fighting over their birthright, and ensured the wife's health was not threatened by too many pregnancies. In countries with population problems, such as China, late marriage is still encouraged.
- A mule's kidney and the urine of eunuchs have been variously recommended for their contraceptive properties.

We have come a long way from those ancient cultures whose women, in despair at endless pregnancies and unwanted children, left newborn babies to die on the hillsides because that was the only way of getting release. This is their story as well as ours.

Scientific Solutions
Potions, Lotions and Enlightened Notions

Science and Medicines

We come now to the stage of our researches known as 'mix-and-match wet', which is the pulling together of diverse contraceptive remedies that consist of pastes and potions concocted to keep babies at bay.

The word 'potion' immediately conjures up a picture of Harry Potter and his chums at Hogwarts gazing glumly at a batch of bubbling test tubes, but the potions used for birth control over the centuries rarely relied on magic. Most had roots in common sense as well as sharp thinking – that's why this chapter also includes 'enlightened notions', as theory drives practice. Interestingly, some of those remedies literally have roots.

That isn't to say that every potion and enlightened notion had a basis in reality. Some of the older ideas in this chapter are so ludicrous they defy belief. In their defence, it should be remembered that they date from times when there was total medical ignorance.

We should also bear in mind that, where ancient remedies were clearly based on science, it is unlikely that the doctors and midwives who prescribed the medicine understood the science. As already mentioned, it was not until the nineteenth century that doctors worked out that it is not just sperm that makes a child, but the fusion of sperm with an egg or ovum.

The bright sparks featured in this section relied on their eyes and ears and carried out their own experiments to get results – results that they could measure, but not always explain.

The Ancient Egyptians

Hubble bubble toil and trouble… 'Here you are, love, stick this in your fanny and it'll do the trick, it's just a bit of crocodile dung mixed with various bits and pieces. Mmmm, smells good, doesn't it?'

If that sounds unlikely, think again because it's precisely what the good women of ancient Egypt were doing to keep conception at bay. How do we know? Because we've got the proof – in writing. And what's more, the oldest evidence, the Ebers Papyrus, was found stored, most appropriately, between the legs of a mummy.

The Ebers Papyrus dates from 1552 BC and, once rescued from its comfortable lodgings, was sold first to a farmer called Edwin Smith who then sold it on to the German Egyptologist, Georg Ebers, from whom it gets its name. Ebers immediately recognized its enormous historical significance – included in the 110 pages of medical information are not only the first recorded cases of diabetes but, also, a recipe for a contraceptive pessary.

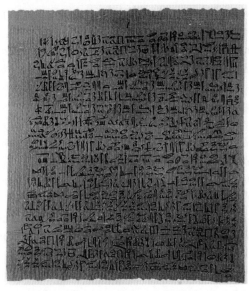

The Ebers Papyrus confirmed the extraordinary medical advances of the ancient Egyptians, for whom contraception was a primary concern.

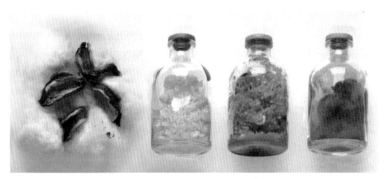

Seed wool, honey, dates and acacia were ingredients used by Egyptian women to make pessaries during the time of Tutankhamun. Honey, a favourite for its medical properties, features regularly in ancient formulae.

Women, we're told, would pound together dates, acacia bark and a bit of honey to make a paste, then steep a piece of seed wool in the mixture and place it in the vulva. Bizarre as this sounds, the pessary – an oozing tablet that was popped inside the vagina before intercourse – would have had some effect because, as it warms, acacia turns into lactic acid, which is a recognized spermicide. It is another example of ancient Egyptian brilliance and not just an old mummy's tale.

In 1889, while excavating at Lahun, the explorer Flinders Petrie discovered the Kahun Papyrus, which dated back to the reign of Pharaoh Amenemhet II (*c.* 1932–1826 BC) . The papyrus contained thirty-four paragraphs of text on female gynaecology, including a suggestion that to diagnose a pregnancy one should place an onion bulb deep in the patient's vagina. If the smell carried to her nose, it meant she was with child.

Another intriguing line from the Kahun Papyrus refers to a pregnant woman with toothache. The suggested remedy is that she should have the urine of a donkey that had just given birth poured over her. Equally curious is the recipe within its pages for a contraceptive pessary, although it does not carry the same weight as that in the Ebers Papyrus. The main ingredients of this pessary were crocodile dung mixed with honey and some sour milk.

Originally, the preferred dung of the Egyptians was that of the elephant, and anyone who has seen the size of the average dropping would calculate that each bowel movement probably provided as many as thirty pessaries. But the paucity of elephants in Egypt made it hard to come by, so they went from using the faeces of the ultimate herbivore to the stools of the ultimate carnivore – the crocodile. There is no record of the difference this made, but it must be assumed that the odour of a meat-eater's pooh is not as wholesome as that of a vegetarian.

The Aztecs also had a thing about pooh, recommending eagle excrement mixed with the plant calabash. It has been reported that, later in history, Tibetan women were given oral contraceptives that included excrement from the Dalai Lama, but evidence is hard to track down. So let's stick with Egypt...

The Ebers Papyrus is now under lock and key at the University of Leipzig, and the Kahun Papyrus is stored at University College, London. Both provide pointers as to how Cleopatra (69–30 BC) managed to seduce with such impunity while only having two

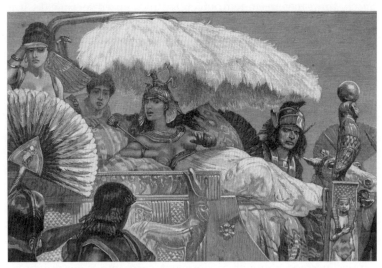

Whether Cleopatra, Queen of Egypt from 47 BC to 30 BC, ever tried out elephant dung as a contraceptive method is one of history's secrets, but it is known that she had a son with Julius Caesar, and later conceived twins with Mark Anthony.

pregnancies. First, she bore a son by the Roman Emperor, Caesar, whom she named Ptolemy IV Caesar; and then she had twins by the love of her life (and Caesar's right-hand man), Mark Anthony, a girl and a boy, named Cleopatra Selene and Alexander Helios.

Alas, it all ended tragically with the two great lovers running away only to find themselves parted. He killed himself and she locked herself away. Still, at least, thanks to family planning at that time, she left only three children without a mother.

The Egyptians must also be credited with inventing the first form of condom. The earliest drawing of a condom, which dates back 3,000 years, is from Egypt, though it isn't so much the device one notices in the illustration as the size of the member it sheaths (see page 94).

Old Eastern Remedies

Not long after, the Indians were making pastes for both internal and external use. The famed first-century physician Charaka, whose natural methodology provides a basis for much Ayurvedic thinking even today, recommended putting cotton soaked in oil from the neem tree inside the vagina for fifteen minutes before intercourse.

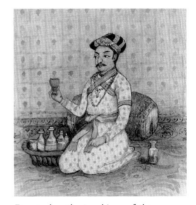

Today, neem is used to deter agricultural pests, and is also an ingredient in toothpastes and skin creams. It has been used in India for 4,000 years. Recent experiments on the subcontinent found that neem oil can kill sperm in under a minute, and ways of manufacturing it for contraceptive use are currently being researched. So Charaka, whose beliefs and philosophy stem from the argument that the body is a self-healing organism striving constantly for perfect balance, was spot on.

Even today, the teachings of the first-century Indian physician Charaka form the basis for Ayurvedic healing; and he was certainly astute in recommending neem oil as a contraceptive.

Later, with the advent of the *Kama Sutra* – the great methodology of love and lovemaking written by Vatsayana in the fourth century AD – there was a move towards oral contraception.

As his writings and investigations into sexuality became more intensive, Vatsayana concluded that if women ate the kadamba fruit with honey a few days after the end of a period (the kadamba tree, as chance would have it, has heart-shaped leaves) they would enjoy short-term sterility and, therefore were less likely to conceive while engaged in vigorous coupling.

Given the many awkward sexual positions mooted in Vatsayana's great masterpiece – which includes sections on secretions and size, on aphrodisiacs, foreplay and technique, and information on how to do it from just about every angle and in every orifice possessed by both partners – one imagines conception was the least of the woman's worries: 'Eh, love, would you mind untangling my leg from the chandelier before all the blood runs to my head?'

Another fruit that has been taken for hundreds of years by the women of the Indian subcontinent, including Sri Lanka, is the papaya. Legend had it that a papaya a day kept the babies at bay and, amazingly, it has been found to be true. An enzyme in the fruit called papain interacts with body hormones to prevent conception, and women still use it as a backup when nothing else is available. Papaya is also said to destabilize the making of sperm, so it can work both ways.

Other plants suggested for contraceptive purposes in olden times were the seed of the red lotus, palm leaves, molasses (unrefined sugar syrup), palasa (Flame of the Forest) and salmoli (cotton tree) flowers.

Less impressive, though, is an ancient Indian suggestion that if a man took the powder of the herb *curcuma longa*, or turmeric as the cooks among us know it, and mixed it with goat's urine, he need only swallow it to be sterile for the duration of coitus.

One cannot help thinking that the turmeric, if not the Billy Goat Gruff wee, would stain the mouth yellow. You wouldn't want to kiss that man, would you? And yet urine regularly pops up in old recipes for all manner of ills. Even today, there is a school of thought that believes drinking fresh urine in the morning boosts the constitution.

Contemporary personalities who admit to having dabbled include the actress Sarah Miles, the entertainer Rolf Harris and the musician and producer Brian Eno. While Madonna allegedly recommends peeing in the shower for keeping athlete's foot at bay. Three million Chinese a day drink their own urine.

In ancient China, urine would have been considered far more benign than the actual potions drunk by some desperate women – they often died or suffered natural sterilization as a result of ingesting lead and mercury to ward off pregnancy.

But these and similar horror stories did nothing to stop women the world over from imbibing any potion that could either prevent a pregnancy, or destroy it – because to them the alternative was even worse.

The Greeks and Romans

Let's move to Athens, where the unfortunately named Soranus was dispensing advice to second-century Greeks who'd given up on the old-fashioned option of homosexuality as a form of birth control. One of the ideas later recovered from Soranus's celebrated textbook, *On Gynecology*, was for the man to divest himself of his sperm by leaping 'with the heels to buttocks for the sake of expulsion'.

The idea is both bizarre and funny, but Soranus, who trained in Alexandria and settled in Rome, from whence he dispatched his ideas around the ancient world, was not a quack. His book tells us that even then, babies born up to eight weeks early were capable of survival. He also offered practical contraceptive advice to those who didn't want babies in any shape or form. One of these solutions resulted in the greatest strike rate in contraceptive history before the invention of the Pill.

Initially, Soranus made the equivalent of contraceptive sponges for his women patients by steeping soft wool balls in the juices of acidic fruits and nuts. Up to forty recipes are listed in *On Gynecology*. He placed these sponges deep inside the cervix to neutralize sperm. But then he started experimenting with a local plant: silphium. He started giving women diluted silphium on a regular basis and found that it stopped conception – just like that.

Silphium, a giant member of the fennel family, came under such demand that stocks went down. Consequently, it became so expensive that only the richest could afford it. The Greeks were

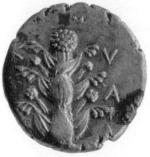

so impressed with silphium that they celebrated it by casting coins with the plant on the back. Within three hundred years, silphium had been harvested to extinction.

But there were other solutions down on the farm. A fellow Greek, Theophrastus, noticed that cattle eating wild carrots were less likely to conceive. Hippocrates – he of the Hippocratic oath taken by doctors the world over – took that intelligence one step further and suggested women wishing to avoid pregnancy should start chewing wild carrot seeds.

An ancient Greek coin showing the plant silphium, which, reputedly, was so successful as a contraceptive that it was farmed to extinction.

Known here as 'Queen Anne's lace' and used later by European midwives, wild carrot seeds have been proven to prevent or abort pregnancy in rats. They are still used as a natural contraceptive remedy by people in the West.

No kitchen garden? Then help could be found in the kitchen cupboard. Aristotle noted a number of women who rubbed olive oil into the cervix as a contraceptive, thus impeding the travel of the man's sperm. Olive oil was used as a deterrent in England as recently as the 1930s.

Archaeologists digging over the remains of the great Roman city Pompeii, which was buried under a sea of hot lava by the eruption of Mount Vesuvius, found the tools of abortion – dilators and curettes – among the priceless mosaics, pots and amulets.

More commonly, though, people looked to nature for the answers. A favourite contraceptive of Roman good-time girls was the insertion of a pessary made of pomegranate peelings. But across the water, Soranus was warning that inserting overpoweringly pungent agents could cause women to suffer internal ulceration.

Pomegranate is still used in the east for its contraceptive properties. The seeds contain a natural oestrogen and supposedly works in a similar way to the Pill. The Egyptian, Razes, had a recipe for a pessary that included the pith of a pomegranate mixed with animals' earwax, cabbage and whitewash. It has been suggested that, given the probable location of the Garden of Eden being somewhere in the Middle East, the apple given to Eve by Adam may well have been a pomegranate.

Other Ancient Remedies

The Israelites introduced two new ideas that continue to form the backbone of female hygiene and birth control even today. They created the tampon. It was made by wrapping a herb-soaked sea sponge in silk, and attaching a string to it for easy removal. Sea sponge, which in those days was harvested by semi-naked divers, was the forerunner of the modern contraceptive sponge (see pages 63–5).

So desperate were women in those times to avoid pregnancy that they would swallow almost anything, including copper sulphate and animal parts, alongside the known favourites such as pennyroyal tea, a known abortifacient made famous in a song by the rock band Nirvana: *'Sit and drink pennyroyal tea/ Distill the life that's inside of me.'*

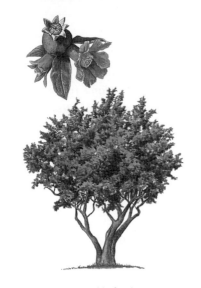

Pomegranate, a visibly fertile fruit bursting with seeds, has, conversely, properties that destabilize the actions of human seeds intent on procreation.

Pennyroyal in the form of tea has been used historically as an abortifacient. Yet, even recently, a young American woman died from taking too much in an attempt to abort a fetus.

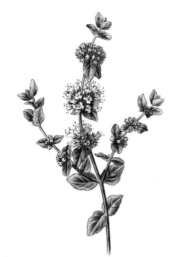

The first evidence of the insertion of a foreign body into the cervix itself actually comes from the Arabs – and was used on camels during long trading journeys. Female camels had stones put into the uterus to stop them conceiving, and this is where the principle of the coil started (see pages 45–58).

Funnily enough, camels these days have a problem reproducing. They have a limited libido, and rutting can go on for hours, running the risk of one or other partner getting bored and wandering off. Male camels tend to leak a lot of semen in the wrong direction. There are, therefore, various schemes in which dromedary camels are being artificially inseminated, and also one where semen is being collected by getting males to rut with a dummy female; the camel equivalent of the blow-up doll. But back to people…

Later practitioners of this contraceptive method experimented by placing glass and metal shapes inside the cervix to prevent pregnancy, but this practice did not supersede herbal remedies, which were easier to administer and to understand.

Nonetheless, the daftest myths continued. In India, a favoured abortion remedy was to sit over a steaming pot of onions or to burn margosa wood and smoke out the genital tract – no

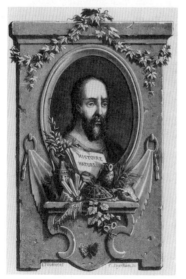

more crazy, presumably, than drinking gin and sitting in a hot bath or rooting around with a knitting needle (see pages 133–6).

In the first millennium, Pliny the Elder (*c.* AD 23–79) claimed that removing two worms from a particular spider, wrapping them in deer skin and attaching them to a woman's body would act as a preventative if completed before dawn.

*Pliny the Elder (*c.* AD 23–79) enters the contraception hall of fame for the most outlandish idea of all time: it involved worms, spiders and deerskin.*

Someone else suggested a woman should spit into the open mouth of a frog three times and this would strike her barren for a year. Later, of course, they changed the story and said she should kiss the frog and that way, at least, she'd meet a prince.

Medieval Europe

In medieval Europe, there was some understanding of herbs and their properties. Midwives took on the role of birth-control practitioners: a practice that had to be carried out on the quiet as any form of intervention was against the teachings of the Catholic Church.

As with ancient experts, midwives had learned about natural remedies through trial and error – potions were passed down through the years from mother to daughter. If they could not limit a woman's fertility, they could mix up a brew that could cause miscarriage. Herbs used included stock garden plants, such as sage, thyme, parsley and rosemary, as well as more complex additives: artemisia, juniper, aloe, willow, cypress, rue and squirting cucumber.

The appositely named squirting cucumber gets its name because the fruit of the plant forcibly ejects the seeds when it ripens, expelling with them a thick juice that dries to become elaterium, a diuretic that also causes chronic nausea and vomiting. It is highly poisonous and those women who administered it to clients had presumably refined their skills at some human cost.

But any help was better than none. Unfortunately, in the climate of religious fervour that accompanied the medieval age and the era that followed it, the skills of the midwives in manipulating the human body left them open to accusations of witchcraft and the dark arts. Between 1450 and 1700, Western Europeans started burning so-called witches – virtually all women – at the stake. King James I of England (1566–1625) – he of the King James Bible – is quoted as saying: 'The more women, the more witches.'

In Italy, the I Benandanti fertility sect had symbolic duels with local witches in the nearby forests. The I Benandanti would wave sticks of fennel in the air while the witches had sorghum stalks as their weapon of choice. Fennel is supposed to prevent natural abortion, while sorghum has abortifacient properties. It would be funny if it weren't for the outcome.

Some may argue, however, that the Benandanti (which means do-gooders) got their come-uppance. They were later branded as witches themselves, and persecuted. Today, their descendants openly associate themselves with white (benign) witchcraft.

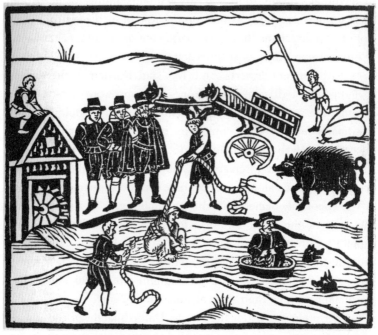

The persecution of women believed to be witches saw the State and God taking over as guardians of women's virtue and fertility. Much expertise was lost and women were forced to put their bodies into the care of male doctors or 'quacks'.

It has been suggested that the total number of witch-burnings carried out in medieval Europe was at least 500,000 and possibly ran into millions. At least one-third of these so-called witches are said to have been midwives.

This huge loss of numbers and skills had a debilitating effect on birth control. The male doctors of the time had little experience in this area, and the women of Europe were literally thrown back into the Dark Ages. One of the silliest ideas doing the rounds at the time was that a woman could prevent pregnancy if she swallowed a bee.

So here they were – 3,000 years on from the Ebers Papyrus and in a state of greater ignorance than the ancient Egyptians because those who had medical qualifications were not interested in what was essentially a women's issue, and those who were interested and had the knowledge were being killed for attempting medical intervention.

Modern Times

But by the late nineteenth century, with the free-thinkers demanding that women should have access to contraception (see pages 76–7) pessaries returned to the scene when a chemist in London's East End, a W. J. Rendell, offered women pessaries of cocoa butter and quinine. They were such a hit that he had to manufacture them full-time.

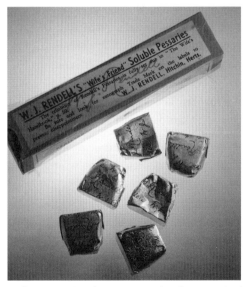

These days, cocoa butter is a popular moisturizer, but for women in the 1890s it was a major ingredient in contraceptive pessaries that were inserted into the vagina before intercourse.

It's interesting that potions and lotions are no longer considered when advocating contraceptive care. This is mainly because contraception, largely, can be dispensed in pill form. Lotions and potions have also been transmogrified into what we call spermicides – gels and creams inserted inside the vagina – to do the same job as acacia or crocodile dung though, hopefully, with less mess and greater success (see pages 72–4).

The pessary has been replaced either with barrier methods or IUDs (Intra-uterine Devices). And the enlightened notions have now moved on to a new level of contraceptive – and conceptive – aid with such technical wizardry as ovulation-testing kits and the morning-after pill, which comes to the rescue when you've had unprotected sex (see page 138).

We now know that emptying the bladder after sex cuts down the chances of getting a bladder infection from the bump and the grind. And, equally, we have learnt that douching or jumping up and down to expel sperm does nothing to minimize the risk of pregnancy.

Our forebears were open to all sorts of ideas because the need for birth control was pressing. What's surprising is not how many of their ideas were off-the-wall, but how many of them had a basis in scientific fact. These days, if there is ignorance it comes from people not having access to the right information, and not because the information that is available is hypothetical. Given all the pitfalls they faced, the ancients did a pretty good job.

Magic Tricks
Abstinence, Amulets and the Snip

Spells and Charms

When trawling through diverse cultural solutions to the age-old problem of staving off babies, it's sometimes difficult to find a common thread.

This chapter is devoted to inevitable logic: indisputable truths about fertility based on human behaviour; the most obvious being that if a man and woman have unprotected penetrative sex they run the risk of having babies.

But it also looks at the illogical solutions. Alongside the practice of leaving well alone, other methods have been devised over the ages to let you bonk yourself barmy with nothing to stave off the inevitable but a magic charm.

The tenuous link between ruthlessly efficient abstinence and the wearing of totems to ward off conception is that external forces, such as God and Nature, have often been called on to justify both.

The lore of amulets looked to earthly forces and the elements and the mythic properties of certain beasts for justification. The logic of abstinence, and derivatives thereof, looked to God and politics for its raison d'être. As such, both methods are enshrined in the theology and ideology of controlling bodies.

Here, we look at the influence of both Church and State: with the caveat that

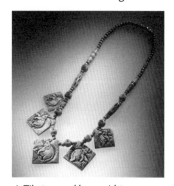

A Tibetan necklace said to have contraceptive powers.

pronouncing on the moral rights and wrongs of methodology, and how it has been administered or enforced, is beyond the concerns of this book. So, let us juxtapose the divine and the meticulous with the lupine and the ridiculous.

Abstinence – Doing It but not Doing 'It'

In the first chapter of this book, we paid homage to the success rate of our forebears in preventing pregnancy. Many of the methods that they hit upon through brilliance or careful observation did have some success, and some methods were almost foolproof. But not all… and I'll come to the beaver testicles shortly.

Other ideas, though utterly rational, were also perverse in the way that they side-stepped sexual pleasure and need: abstinence, for example. Some cultures sought only to find alternative solutions for men – which is why homosexuality was promulgated as a suitable vehicle for getting your rocks off.

Abstinence is the most obvious form of contraception: no sex means no babies. But as we have discovered time and again in our own lives – it doesn't work. An obvious example is with priests of the Roman Catholic Church, all of whom take a vow of celibacy. It has not stopped endless numbers of them from fathering children…

The difficulty in following the path of righteousness was also acknowledged in ancient times. There is the famous story, now disputed by Papal scholars, of Pope Joan, who got the top job in the Vatican by calling herself John. Joan allegedly gave birth to a baby at a roadside while holding the Papacy. This just goes to show that any method that is totally dependent on human beings acting against their natural instincts is open to failure.

You only have to look at the letters in the problem pages of today's magazines to come across a glut of excuses for unplanned heat-of-the-moment sexual intercourse: 'we got carried away', 'it just happened', 'one minute we were kissing and then…'.

Remember Boris Becker, an otherwise sensible married man, who inexplicably threw himself into a one-minute encounter with a waitress in a hotel broom cupboard? He lost his wife and ended up with an unplanned child and a lifetime of child support. Control goes through the window when lust enters by the door.

So, if abstinence poses a difficulty, what's the next best option? For the ancient Greeks, they of the Priapic statues, the answer was same-sex sex. They adopted homosexuality as an acceptable alternative. And the Romans, while not supporting it in legal channels, considered it a plausible option.

But, obviously, unless you're gay by inclination, this isn't the best of substitutes, and the wife might start to get a tad annoyed as you embark on yet another night out with the boys. So it was, then, that the generic use of homosexuality as a contraceptive aid faded out within the very cultures that had promoted it, and was never really considered by others.

There is, of course, a slightly more gratifying half-way option: *coitus interruptus* or withdrawal – the man pulling out of the woman before the moment of ejaculation. It doesn't sound very edifying, but there are those who've made a fortune in the porn industry for their skill at pulling out in time for the classic 'come shot'.

Unfortunately, for those dependent on the Bible for guidance, the experience of Onan – who angered God by pulling out of his sister-in-law and spilling his seed on the ground – suggested to most Christians that to indulge in *coitus interruptus* was a sin. (And no, Onan wasn't being a bad boy by playing with his brother's wife. The brother had died and it was a local custom that he should take over and produce babies with her.)

Getting swiftly tarred by the same brush, all other types of sexual gratification were also judged to be sinful. Masturbation, the spilling of seed with no partner present, is considered a form of onanism because the purpose of seed is procreation.

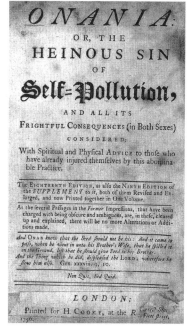

In Western cultures, many young boys grew up believing that masturbation was a sin for which they would be struck down by the wrath of God. This notice from 1722 also encompasses masturbation by women.

Prostitutes and STDs

So, if abstinence is difficult and withdrawal is unacceptable, what are the other options? In Europe, the obvious solution was not to give up on sex but to have it with women of ill repute. Prostitutes, presumably, had recourse to herbal remedies in the event of conception. And, even if they didn't, they had the added benefit of not having a reputation to sully any further. What's more, they couldn't spoil the man's life with an unwanted, illegitimate child. They also helped minimize the risk to his wife's life by making it less likely that she would get 'in the family way'.

In other words, at a time when there was no fail-safe method of contraception (and the maternal death rate was one per 154 live births), men went to prostitutes to discharge their need and their seed rather than risk impregnating their partners.

The downside of this bright idea was that large numbers of men, from kings to potboys, contracted venereal diseases. The most rampant of these was syphilis, which appears in the form of small blisters similar to herpes, but has far more fearful repercussions if untreated. In pre-penicillin days – that is, before the mid-twentieth century – there was no real cure for syphilis and sufferers would experience fevers, fatigues, hair-loss, tissue-loss, paralysis and heart disease.

Even royalty was affected by what William Shakespeare (1564–1616) referred to as 'the French Disease' in *Henry V* – a Saxe-Coburg forebear of Henry V's wife, Katherine of France, shot himself to escape the pain of tuberculosis aggravated by venereal disease. For the rich, the preferred alternative to using prostitutes was to engage in affairs with actresses who were sexually open but serially monogamous. One of the most famous of these was Nell Gwynn (1650–87), who referred to the child she had by King Charles II (1630–85) as 'the little bastard'.

The boy, also called Charles, was one of thirteen children the king sired with his various mistresses – though it isn't clear whether or not his queen, Catherine of Braganza, was happy about this. When Charles heard Nell refer to their son as a 'bastard', he immediately made the youth Duke of St Albans.

For those men without recourse to the lively ladies of the stage, syphilis was a terrible legacy. Inevitably, large numbers of men unwittingly passed the disease on to their wives, and, via them, on to their legitimate children, who suffered bone abnormalities, corneal inflammation, arthritis, peg-shaped teeth and mental abnormality.

Syphilis is still around today, but if caught in the early stages, it can be blitzed with a course of antibiotics. The disease even gets a mention in the popular TV series, *Buffy the Vampire Slayer:*

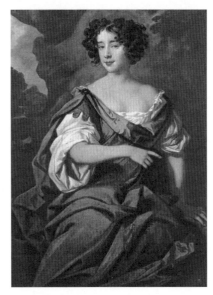

Nell Gwynn called herself 'the Protestant whore' and was one of a number of women used by male royalty to protect their wives from serial pregnancy.

XANDER: You know what? I think my syphilis is clearing right up.
BUFFY: And they say romance is dead.

Romance is not dead, but sexual trust has been eroded in recent years. With the spread of HIV, modern lovers have been forced to face similar ugly truths about sexually transmitted diseases to those of their predecessors. The virus, and its potentially fatal consequences if it progresses to full-blown AIDS, has forced the modern-day public to consider the consequences of unprotected sex.

Today, a lot of people associate the wearing of lapel ribbons with the huge HIV/AIDS-awareness campaign that was launched in the 1990s. Suddenly, we were all wearing a little bow pinned to our clothing to help raise consciousness and funds for those who were affected. But the idea of donning a lapel ribbon predates HIV by over 100 years, and even then it was associated with sexuality and sexual behaviour.

In 1885, whoring American men became a new target for the Women's Temperance Movement – an organization set up to get men out of public houses and return them to the redemptive fold of a Christian God. The Temperance Movement, in a bid to cut down on sexual practices that left innocent women susceptible to hideous lurgies, urged men to wear white ribbons on their lapels as a sign of monogamy and sexual purity. In its own way, the wheel has come full circle.

Lest we forget, let's take a moment out here to remind ourselves that some barrier methods, such as the condom and Femidom, are not just contraceptives, they also protect men and women against sexually transmitted diseases (see pages 91–110). The number of adults with syphilis and HIV attending clinics that treat such diseases is rising each year. So, use contraception for safe sex as well as for birth control. You have been told.

So, we have abstinence, withdrawal, homosexuality and prostitution as alternatives to pregnancy. More recently, since the nineteenth-century discovery that a woman contributes an egg to the fertilization process, we have been given the 'rhythm method'. Put broadly, a woman with a regular menstrual cycle ovulates on the fourteenth day of her cycle. At that point, there is a three-day window of intense fertility. If she avoids copulation around that time, she can – hopefully – avoid pregnancy. The problem with this method is that eggs can hang around a little longer, as can old sperm. Therefore, it is not foolproof.

For women with more erratic cycles, the daily taking of temperature can tell you when ovulation is happening, because your body temperature increases. Again, this is nowhere near foolproof.

Ovulation kits (see pages 147–8) have been developed that pinpoint the hormonal surge that heralds fertility (see pages 122–3); but these kits are recommended as fertility aids rather than as contraceptives due to the variations in each woman's cycle. However, it must be said in their favour that, along with all the other possibilities open to women in terms of natural remedies, these remedies clearly worked to some extent – in the West, at least.

Bizarre Magic and Practices

One doesn't need to reiterate how unreliable all and any of these practices can be but, even so, when compared to some of the more bizarre beliefs that predate a lot of them, they're positively brilliant.

Soranus, the Greek medic, has been mentioned in this tome for his more scientific approach, including recipes for vaginal pessaries and the discovery of silphium (see pages 25–6) – but among his seriously weird ideas was the suggestion that a woman should hold her breath just as the man is about to ejaculate, thus contracting the os – the entrance to the womb – then squat on the floor with her legs wide apart and 'sneeze' out his deposit.

A Persian scholar suggested a similar method involving the woman hopping backwards several times while maintaining her squat. Easy!

At weddings in sixteenth-century Yugoslavia, the bride put an open padlock inside her bodice and then took as many steps as she wished to have childless years. Having done that, be it two or twenty, she closed the padlock, had intercourse with her consort in the usual way, and truly believed her little ritual would keep the ankle-biters at bay.

And then, of course, there was the legendary chastity belt, which wasn't just a birth-control device but enforced abstinence and fidelity, thereby preventing the conception of someone else's baby. It was bought by married men who were about to go to war or hurry off on other urgent business, and was locked into place on their wives' bodies as they departed.

The chastity belt was effectively a pair of metal knickers, though it was also available in bone and ivory. The gusset had a hole big

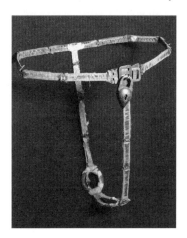

The chastity belt: fact or fantasy? Fearsome-looking iron belts with locks are displayed in museums, but no evidence has yet been found to suggest they were commonly used.

enough for urination but not big enough for a finger to be inserted…

A number of chastity belts have been unearthed and examined by historians, including one that, ostensibly, dates back to the seventeenth century and was found on the remains of a corpse in Austria. However, there is still uncertainty about their usage, how common they were, and on whom they were used.

One such belt, displayed in a French museum, looks a little like a thong and has a cut-out star at the front. It's very pretty. The area covered by the metal is about the size and shape of the modern Brazilian bikini wax, front and back. It thins in the middle of the gusset, near the urethra, and has a small hole for the anus. Yikes! Again, though, one can see the logic here: if a woman can't actually access her private parts, nobody else has a hope of doing so either.

How, though, does one explain the proliferation of *testes* as a form of useful contraceptive? Think about this: a form of birth control during medieval times was for a woman to be given weasel testicles to hang on her thigh. If, for any reason, she found this difficult, another solution was to amputate the weasel's foot and wear it round her neck as an amulet: the weasel's footloose and the woman's fancy free…

Back to old bollocks: Canadian women living in New Brunswick used to brew up beaver testicles with alcohol to make a contraceptive drink. Staying in the same anatomical area, another medieval favourite was to create an amulet from a hare's anus.

The hare, of course, is a creature often connected with folklore. There is something about its stillness and open, staring eyes that inspires fantastic imaginings – both good and bad. The hare is believed to have been introduced to Britain by the Romans. Only two types exist: the lowlands brown hare and the blue mountain hare. A hare's foot was said to ward off rheumatism and Boudicca (d. 62 AD) considered them a portent of tribal victory.

Conversely, the term 'hare lip' comes from the Middle Ages when people believed that a woman who saw a hare while pregnant would give birth to a child with this deformity, as the hare was seen to be a tool of the devil. In Germany, children believe Easter eggs are laid by hares. This myth is believed to stem from the plover, which makes its nest on the ground near hare's forms, which are the hollows in the ground where hares sit. Should the hare leave, the plover moves its nest into the form to hatch its babies there.

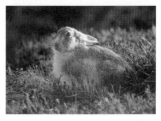

The thought of the hare's anus being removed and turned into a neck ornament gives a whole new spin to the notion of potted hare. But the belief that certain beings or substances contain medicinal or magical properties to ward off particular threats or conditions is, of course, nothing new.

Hares feature frequently in all mythology. One of the most peculiar ideas was to use a hare's anus to minimize fertility.

Even today, Christians wear medallions featuring St Christopher to help promote safe travel, while Hindus and Buddhists have strands of prayer reel tied round their wrists to ward off evil. Sufferers of arthritis wear copper bangles, whereas if I ever I feel a sty coming up on my eye I rub gold against it and it goes away – or at least appears to.

Practitioners of alternative therapies commonly hand out everything from scented oils to crystals, claiming that they have power over our well-being and environment – and we believe them. So it's hardly surprising that in the darker ages, without the benefit of the scientific knowledge that we have today, people had good reason to believe in external forces holding power over internal impulses or workings. That's why, when women got told to soak a cloth in menstrual blood, wrap it in a piece of flax lint and carry it around to ward off pregnancy, they did it.

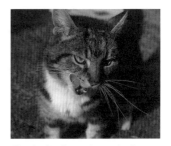

It's also why cats played a big part in past contraceptive methods. Cats have had spiritual associations since ancient times, when the Egyptians believed male cats descended from the Sun God, Ra, and female cats represented the solar eye. They even mummified cats and buried them in special cemeteries. But in medieval England, the cat was used more practically as a birth-control device. Their desiccated livers were

If only the domestic cat had contraceptive properties… In ancient times cats' livers were worn in amulet form to ward off fertility.

made into amulets, as were the bone shards of black cats; maybe that's why black cats are still considered to be lucky now.

There were also the standard herb amulets and, interestingly, a belief that if you circled a place where a pregnant wolf had urinated, you would become temporarily infertile. Drinking a wolf's pee was another remedy. It seems laughable, but I couldn't find any research to say it doesn't work. After all, if passive smoking can cause asthma; and the smell of a peanut can cause a fatal allergic reaction; and the fumes from lead-free petrol are carcinogenic; who's to say wolf's urine *doesn't* let off a chemical that might affect, for example, progesterone levels?

Since the age of the Aztecs, Mexican women have eaten a wild yam, the *cabeza de negro*, to ward off pregnancy. Today, that same yam supplies the synthetic progesterone that is the mainstay of the contraceptive pill (see page 115).

Sterilization

But if you're set on a tougher route, and even the tiniest risk is too much, the most sensible option on offer is sterilization. Should sterilization be considered in a book about the history of birth control when it doesn't control fertility but brings fertility to an end electively? It's a hard call, but as the thinking behind such decisions must necessarily take in the other options it has a limited place.

Male sterilization, vasectomy, is effectively the sacking of sperm; it does not affect ejaculation, as some people assume. The man still releases semen, but the semen does not contain those tadpole-shaped buggers that cause all the trouble. It's a simple enough operation involving the cutting of the *vas deferens*, the sperm duct, so it can no longer feed into the penis. This method requires only an out-patient visit and is almost totally foolproof. It can, however, cause a little discomfort for up to two weeks.

That said, compared to childbirth, it's the difference between cutting your finger and amputating an arm: unless you use the traditional Aboriginal system as described by J. G. Garson in 1894. Garson, a doctor who studied the tribes of Australia, reported that sterilization was carried out by making an incision in the scrotum and severing the urethra, so that urine and semen would, thereafter, seep out of the new hole. Yow!!

India boasts the largest number of men with vasectomies: 13 million volunteered for the process between 1967 and 1973. But even that wasn't enough to help keep India's birth rate down. At one point the Government of Mrs Indira Gandhi came under serious international pressure when, in a bid to stem the country's burgeoning population, she brought in a law enforcing sterilization on men who had already had three children. Following this enforced sterilization, the number of men who had had the snip in India jumped to 22 million between 1973 and 1977, but the policy was dropped due to its unpopularity.

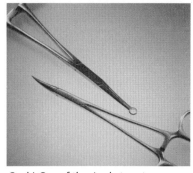

Ouch! One of the simplest contraceptive procedures is the vasectomy – but it's the point of no return.

In China, alongside the one-child law (see page 131), sterilization is offered free to any man or woman who already has a child.

Castration

If any kind of enforced sterilization sounds awful, imagine what it was like to undergo enforced castration. The removal of a man's testicles at an early age was practised by the Italians to turn young male sopranos into old male sopranos. Castration prevented boys' voices from breaking at a time when only men performed on the stage, but it also ensured they were never distracted by sex and babies.

It is suggested that later surgical techniques left the *castrati*, as these men were known, able to have sexual relations despite the loss of their testes – so, theoretically, castration can work as a form of contraceptive. It also made the *castrati* incredibly lucky men as the best were revered for their voices and earned vast fortunes: sex, song and money – who's complaining? But there were also hundreds who didn't make it to the top and whose lives were blighted forever.

In Eastern cultures, castrated men called eunuchs were created to guard the harems of their royal masters and provide entertainment, as the lack of male hormone made them something between feminine and masculine. The legendary Syrian queen Semiramis is said to have had all her lovers castrated, to ensure they never pleasured other women. Some say it also prevented a male challenging her power.

For a woman, sterilization can now be done by laparoscopy – that is, through the belly button or through an incision just below it. It's more risky than a vasectomy because it's more invasive. The principle, however, is the same. The surgeon cuts or clips off the connectors to the Fallopian tubes and seals them, thus stopping the passage of eggs to the womb. The failure rate is very low and you have *medical* evidence of your sterility, unlike some poor women documented in the Berlin Papyrus. This ancient Egyptian artefact reports that women were fumigated with hippopotamus dung to test for infertility: if they peed, poohed or farted afterwards they were deemed barren.

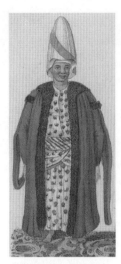

Some Eastern cultures created impotent eunuchs to watch over harems.

If any of the more outlandish ideas in this section have had you giggling, it's woth noting that we have modern ideas that are no less ludicrous. Surveys show that some young people still believe you can't get pregnant if you make love standing up; if you ejaculate near the vagina but not in it; or if you cover the penis with anything going, including clingfilm and sweet wrappers. So what are we to make of these sometimes hard-line and sometimes plain daft options for birth control?

There is little to say beyond the obvious: sexuality even in an age of open discussion and availability of information is complex, because it engages strong emotions that often blind us to the necessary or push us towards any remedy that might help. It remains an area of absolutes – of absolute certainty and, inevitably, absolute confusion.

The Coil
Wired and Sound

The Use of Foreign Bodies

All forms of birth control have antecedents stretching back to ancient times, and the coil or Intra-uterine Device (IUD) is no different.

It does, however, have a much smaller and sketchier history than other methods of birth control. The reasons for this become obvious when you start thinking about it.

Any device that has to be lodged within the uterus will necessarily bring pain, rejection or disease unless the design is so perfect that no nasty little germs can hop on board and use it as a conduit for sneaking inside and causing trouble.

The manner of insertion is also important: how do you organize the drop-off of the alien package in circumstances that guarantee no internal contamination? After all, lodging a foreign body in a sterile environment necessarily hikes the odds in favour of medical failure.

It's a tricky balance to strike and, even in modern times, there have been many problems – including death and disease – associated with the methodology. As a result, the IUD, despite an excellent success rate, does not have a large take-up in the West, although it's popular elsewhere, particularly in China.

What is often forgotten is that, alongside the Pill, the coil is one of the newest forms of birth control. Although it had its forerunners, it was not mooted for mass use until the 1960s. In development terms, it is still very young. Future histories of contraception will mark the coil's recent past as a necessary blip in the evolution of birth control, and that context should be borne in mind.

Foreign Bodies in Our Bodies

The first purported record of the use of an IUD is of Arab merchants putting stones inside the cervix of female camels to prevent pregnancy.

It would obviously be problematic to employ similar tools when dealing with humans, but the principle of the stone in the womb is what inspired the manufacture of the 'coil' – a device that is ninety-nine per cent effective at deflecting sperm and preventing pregnancy.

Stones aside, the principle of the IUD in workable terms, is relatively recent because it took many attempts (and a series of highly publicized problems) for us to reach the stage where IUDs could be said, without equivocation, to work entirely in a woman's favour.

It is one of the great mysteries and wonders of the coil that nobody yet understands how or why it works. It has been suggested that inserting an IUD thickens the mucus at the neck of the cervix so that it forms a repellent plug. If you like, it acts like a bouncer at the door to the womb: throwing out all undesirables in the shape of fast-swimming sperm.

Equally likely is that when womb conditions are not totally favourable the body's natural response is to avoid pregnancy. After all, for the fittest to survive, the body must be primed to produce the best while it is in peak condition. If an egg rolls into the womb and discovers it's going to be fighting for space, then it's clearly less hassle to bail out at the end of the monthly cycle than to stay, put up a fight and risk damage.

Looking at pictures of the coil can be confusing because it isn't a coil at all, but a slightly curved T-shaped object of about 1½ inches (4cm) in length and made out of plastic or copper. However, when the modern coil was first introduced to the market in the 1960s, it looked like a lasso – the rope loop used by cowboys to harness horses. (Interestingly, the female horse, like the female

The term 'coil' comes from the first successful IUD to go into production, the Lippes Loop, but its forerunners and successors come in many different shapes and sizes.

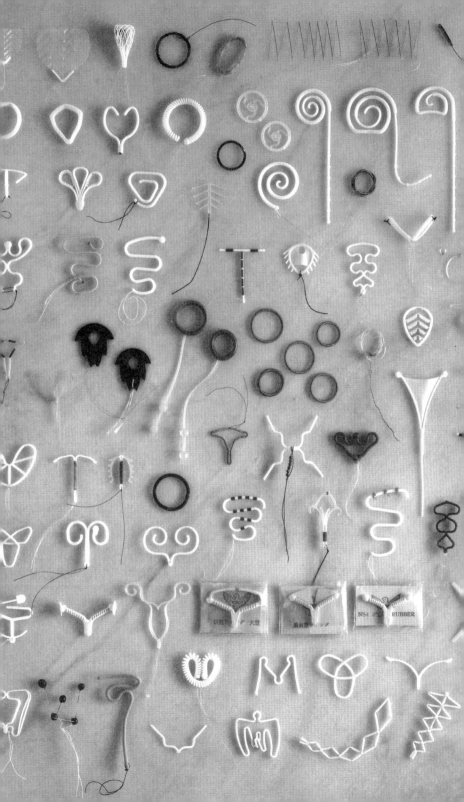

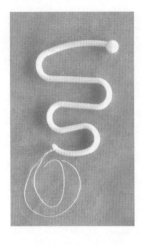

The Lippes Loop resembles a coil of rope, or a lasso, and first came onto the contraceptive market in the 1960s.

human, responds far better to a sexual advance if first prepared through foreplay. In the breeding of racehorses it is quite common for a mare to be licked into action by a 'ringer' – or a 'fluffer' as the female equivalent on porn filmsets is called– before the hired stud is led into the stable to perform a multi-million pound coupling.)

'Lasso' is, however, a singularly unattractive word to apply around human females, and so the device, initially called the loop, became the coil. But before we get to that point, there is some production history that we need to know.

The Legacy of Grafenberg

It was in 1902 that a German doctor, Carl Hollweg, invented a pessary that extended into the womb. Hollweg's device carried too much risk of infection for it to work, but the basic design excited interest. The logic behind the idea was sound.

Within years a fellow countryman, Richard Richter, had built upon Hollweg's thinking, creating a more workable product using bronze rings, which he threaded with silk. The device was too large, however, to be inserted safely into the cervix.

It was in 1929 that Ernst Grafenberg perfected a workable proto-type. The Grafenberg Ring was smaller and made of silver with an unrecorded copper content (copper would later be identified as increasing the effectiveness of the coil).

Unlike Richter's device, Grafenberg's did not have an extruding string (or wick) by which infection and disease could be conducted, and so it went into production. Grafenberg recommended using

The Grafenberg Ring was a major step in the right direction in the search for an IUD that did not cause side effects. Nevertheless, there were problems and it was withdrawn from use.

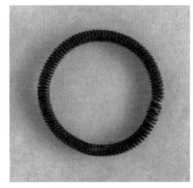

antiseptic during insertion to minimize the chances of pelvic inflammatory disease (PID). Nonetheless, a large number of women suffered from PID, so the inventor went back to the drawing board.

PID has historically been associated with the coil because fitting it provides opportunities for germs to get into the reproductive organs. This can result in excruciating abdominal pain, nausea and vomiting. On the one hand, this is a good thing as it alerts sufferers to the need for help in the form of antibiotics. On the other, if left untreated, it could lead to infertility and increases the chances of a life-threatening ectopic pregnancy, in which the baby grows in the Fallopian tubes.

The most common cause of PID in the twenty-first century is the increase in sexually transmitted infections. Abortions and childbirth also afford opportunities for stray bacteria to worm their way from the warm and wet vaginal canal into the sterile environment of the uterus, which is where the trouble begins. Although the incidence of PID contracted after coil insertion is relatively negligible these days, women are told to be on the lookout for symptoms in the first weeks after a fitting.

Alas, while Grafenberg was rethinking the construction of his ring, events were conspiring against him.

As you will discover in these pages, contraception is a common tool for making the personal political. Attitudes to birth control are tied in with, and have enforced, the position of women in society. The way that the establishment (the Church and the State) has influenced contraception – its research, its existence, its value and its

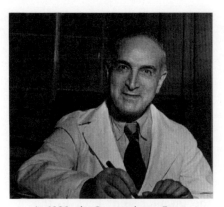

In 1929, the German doctor Ernst Grafenberg (1881–1957) produced a prototype of the modern IUD that should have been foolproof, but wasn't. He is now best known for identifying the G-spot in women.

availability – affects our choices and our decisions.

The IUD was not exempt from the vagaries of dogma: indeed, it was one of the first victims of Hitler's Nazi doctrine. On coming into power in 1933, the Nazis outlawed birth control and offered Aryan couples financial incentives to marry and have children. They stamped out any research that might work against their aim of mass-producing the Aryan line.

As they lost increasing numbers of men during the Second World War (1939–45), the Nazis began to draft laws making it incumbent on a man who had already fathered four children by one woman to go out and father some more by another. However, the idea never made it to statute. Meanwhile, birth-control clinics and sex-reform organizations in a country with a previously high abortion rate were closed down.

For his efforts, Grafenberg was arrested and imprisoned by the Gestapo. His release was only secured after the American family-planning activist Margaret Sanger (see pages 113–25) paid a bounty for him. She invited him to the United States where he worked for her organization before branching out and becoming a man who ultimately gave up on his ring and became instead a sex guru forever associated with female pleasure.

It was Ernst Grafenberg who identified the G-Spot ('G' as in Grafenberg). The G-spot is a ridged point within the vagina, behind the pubic bone, which is supposed to cause frenzied, and often multiple, orgasms, when manipulated. It's a bit like the male prostate gland. One can't help but think it might have been fun having an IUD fitted by the gossamer-fingered doctor.

Grafenberg's exit from his homeland was also vital in reframing the arguments in favour of birth control. Sanger's association with Grafenberg alerted her to the dark side of the eugenics movement. Her motivation in developing birth control was social, based on Malthusian number-crunching, rather than racial. But, through her many associates in Germany, a huge number of whom were Jewish, Sanger grew to see that some doctrines can never be disconnected from politics. However, Sanger also understood that arguing the principle, no matter how high-minded, is fallacious given the bigger picture. This new intelligence provided a much healthier springboard for the launch of her prized organization, the Planned Parenthood Federation, in 1952.

It is, however, ironic that the Nazis, a regime intent on wiping out whole populations on a eugenist agenda, and which used those incarcerated in its death camps as guinea pigs for medical science, forced physicians like Grafenberg to stop research that might have helped them suppress 'inferior' races.

Meanwhile, Grafenberg's work was picked up in Japan, where, in the mid-1930s, Dr Tenrei Ota modified his device and turned out gold and gold-plated rings that appeared to have a better success rate than the Grafenberg Ring. But, again, PID raised its ugly head. Ota was one of the first physicians to fashion an IUD out of plastic. Later, maintaining his pro-choice stand at all stages of life, he became a founder member of the Japan Euthanasia Society.

Ota's research into IUDs, however, was as doomed as his German counterpart's. When Japan joined the Axis coalition, Ota's work was also halted. It would be another decade or two before American medics came up with a winning formula.

In 1962, Jack Lippes, a gynaecologist in Buffalo, New York State picked up on various researches and decided a ring was, well… too round. It was too problematic. He changed the shape, and the Lippes Loop was born – the loop that led to the generic term *coil*, and that actually looks like a lasso.

Lippes realized that you had to have a wick extruding from the entrance to the cervix, otherwise insertion and removal became a real circus. His loop had a filament attached and the device was made of polyethylene – a plastic that's used in everything from carrier bags to bulletproof vests and is non-absorbent, thus making it less likely to become a conduit for germs.

The Lippes Loop became the model for the majority of IUDs inserted into women the world over. By the 1970s, plastic and copper were the materials of choice and there was a proliferation of 'coils' on the market in shapes ranging from loops to 'Y's to 'T's.

The Dalkon Shield

The story doesn't end here with the familiar line: 'and they all lived happily ever after'. The success of the IUD meant pharmaceutical companies were fighting for shares in a highly lucrative market. People started taking short-cuts to get products onto the shelves. And so we come to the story of the infamous Dalkon Shield: a plastic IUD that was hugely popular in the United States during a three-year window in the early 1970s.

Dr Hugh Davis designed the shield for the A. H. Robins company of Richmond, Virginia. It was named because of its shape, and it was generally problematic. The main cause was the wick, which was multifilament rather than single filament and was covered in a polymer that degenerated in the vagina, opening the way for germs to accumulate in the uterus. Within months of going on the market, women were presenting doctors with physical problems.

It would later be suggested that Davis had been slapdash in his researches because he was getting a cut from sales, and that Robins rushed the shield onto the market at a time when the American Food and Drug Administration had no authority over contraception.

Twenty Dalkon Shield users died after suffering septic abortions. these occur when a fetus is not fully expelled during a miscarriage, and the remaining tissue becomes infected, thus inflaming the womb. Before antibiotics, septic abortion was the biggest cause of death in pregnant women the world over, primarily as a result of

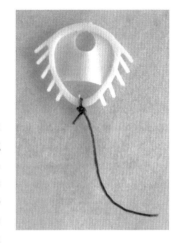

The coil, particularly the Dalkon Shield pictured here, had quite a problematic history. This was mainly because it took numerous attempts to find a wicking system that didn't carry infection to the cervix. The coil now has a clean bill of health.

illegal abortions. Septic abortion also happens when an incubating fetus is attacked by outside germs. It's why, once a pregnant woman's waters have broken she's taken to hospital, as the plug preventing the entry of foreign bodies has been removed and the child must either be extracted or protected.

Users of the Dalkon Shield did not anticipate pregnancy, but there were pregnancies. As they progressed, the womb naturally started to swell and, in doing so, pulled up the infected tail of the device, which arrived in a malevolent flash like the bad fairy at the christening of Sleeping Beauty. The result is well documented…

Hundreds of women were left sterile as a result of infection from the Dalkon Shield. In the catalogue of misadventure that would later be prepared, harrowing cases of miscarriage and hysterectomy were told. Of those women who remained fertile, many suffered other fertility issues triggered by the side effects of this IUD.

The ninety-eight per cent success rate associated with the coil plummeted with the arrival of the Dalkon Shield. Up to half a million women would later claim compensation in what became one of the largest civil law suits of its time. The Claimants Trust paid out up to US$3 billion in compensation in the 1990s, by which time A. H. Robins had filed for bankruptcy. The timing of the case was disastrous for all coil manufacturers.

Ironically, before fashioning the Dalkon Shield for A. H. Robins, Dr Davis had attended a hearing about the risks of oral contraception and spoken against the Pill on health grounds. Yet, as he struggled with the fallout from his research, it was the Pill that topped the birth-control charts. The damage to the coil was irreversible; misinformation ruled the day.

After the Dalkon Shield scare, a lot of fuss was made of the increase in PID among IUD users, though later research suggested that this was as much to do with increased numbers of sexual partners. The Americans stopped prescribing the coil until rigorous new testing procedures had been carried out. At the end of that time, only two devices were approved for use. Meanwhile, the Lippes Loop continued to be successful with women in other parts of the world.

The Coil Today: Pros and Cons

Today, the coil and its variations are not recommended for young people indulging in promiscuous behaviour because they are more likely to suffer sexual infection, and any infection is a risk. Women are swabbed and checked before the coil is approved. It is mainly aimed at those with children and older women who cannot take the Pill.

There are still side effects connected to insertion: there is intermittent bleeding for some weeks afterwards, but the heavy periods previously associated with the coil are no longer a problem. For some women, the coil may cause more painful stomach cramps during menstruation and, albeit rarely, a coil may perforate the womb.

Nonetheless, 100 million women worldwide use the coil without side effects – mostly in China and parts of the developing world. Their lives have been revolutionized because the coil, once dispensed, does not require regular visits to a doctor.

Psychologically, though, it's a big step to have a piece of moulded plastic – more usually the T-shape these days – lodged inside the body on a long-term basis. So, what are the advantages for those women that opt for it?

The first, and most obvious, is also the most important: it gives a woman round-the-clock protection from pregnancy for several years. There's no danger of her forgetting to get (or buy) it, as with the condom; or forgetting to take it, as with the Pill. There's no messing about before and after intercourse, which is inevitable with the cap or the sponge. There's no reliance on the body clock or recourse to good luck, as with the rhythm method and withdrawal methods.

Beyond the moment of insertion, which can occasionally be uncomfortable, there are no visits required to doctors or chemists; no repeat prescriptions and no financial outlay. Occasionally, a coil can fall out and women are taught to check that theirs is secure, but that's about it. Once a coil is inserted, you can forget about it for the next five years.

Before the Coil...

Wicking has been identified as the main cause of failure in the history of the IUD, but this didn't stop practitioners trying to find ways around the problem. At the History of Contraception Museum in Toronto, Canada, there are all manner of IUDs, including one that looks like a shepherd's staff or a ram's curly horn on a stick.

This rather lends itself to a joke about rural farmers and their relationship with ewes, but rams also feature in the study of human sexuality. Up to one in ten rams is gay, and while nobody is yet suggesting that there is a genetic pathway to sexual preferences, the same differences have been found in the hypothalamus of gay rams as in the hypothalamus of gay men.

The collection also includes IUDs fashioned as long-tailed triangles and one with a pattern of open diamonds. Another is studded with gemstones and carved in the shape of a crown. It is believed that in some cultures women had pieces of glass and wood inserted into their wombs to prevent pregnancy.

Another antiquated form of IUD is the wishbone pessary, which looks a bit like a two-pronged paper securer (the one with a round head holding together two prongs that you put through a punched hole and open out like an inverse staple).

With the wishbone pessary, the prongs were aligned and in-geniously held in place with wax. Once inserted into the cervix, the heat from the woman's body melted the wax and the prongs parted

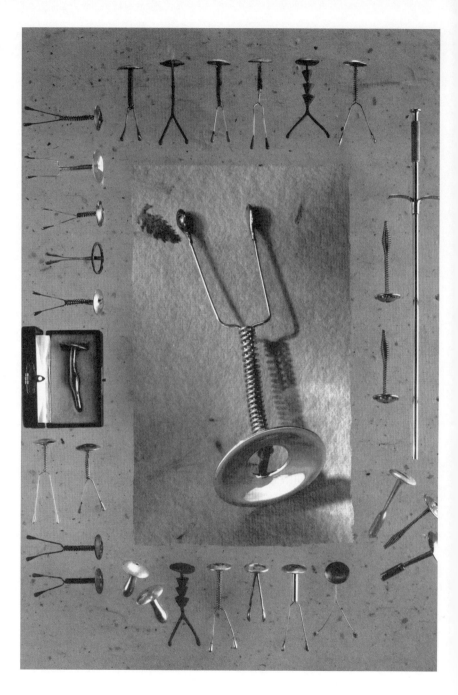

to hold the device in place, the head blocking the entry to the cervix and the prongs disturbing the equilibrium within the womb.

When you consider that the average womb is about the shape and size of a light bulb, you can see how important it is to get the form of the coil, and the mechanism, just right.

After pregnancy, a woman's physiology changes – which is why coils cause less pain and problems for a woman who has had children (see also the diaphragm, pages 65–77).

The wishbone pessary, though ingenious, did not survive the test of time. Thankfully, insertion these days is somewhat simpler: a doctor holds open the vagina with a speculum and slips a straw containing the coil inside the opening of the cervix, which is called the os and looks, literally, like the tip of a penis. The IUD is then pushed out of the straw in a similar manner to that used when employing a tampon applicator.

More recently we've seen the introduction of a super-coil that slowly releases synthetic progesterone into the body, thus increasing its contraceptive properties and limiting menstrual bleeds.

The most common of these is the Mirena Coil, which is not referred to as an IUD but an IUS – an Intra-uterine System – because it has a function beyond the particular. The Mirena Coil has a little store of a synthetic progestin called levonorgestrel, which it releases into the endometrium (the lining of the womb) at a rate of less than an ounce (20mg) a day (see page 123 for more about how proges-terone levels affect fertility).

The Mirena, like all coils, needs replacing every five years but its success rate is phenomenal: 999 to one instead of the usual ninety-eight to two.

Another advantage of the coil, whatever the type, is that it can be used to stop pregnancy after unprotected sex. The insertion of a coil up to five days after intercourse will prevent an egg from

The wishbone pessary was a one-off, and placed itself effectively within the cervix. The prongs were held tightly together by wax, which loosened at body temperature to affix themselves in the womb.

settling in the endometrium. For that reason, many pro-life campaigners disapprove of it, arguing that the coil is not a contraceptive device but an abortifacient: it does not prevent fertilization so much as prevent an egg from embedding and multiplying to a point beyond a few cells.

Whatever the arguments for and against, the very nature of its situation means that coils and their derivatives will always engender debate and occasionally argument. It is still, for all the caveats attached to it (and they seem many only because those around other forms are so few), the most successful and widely used form of global contraception. The spectre of the Dalkon Shield may still haunt women in the Western world, but elsewhere they wouldn't be without the trusty coil.

Cap This
Erecting Barriers . . .

Taking the Hands-on Approach 'Down There'

One of the worst indignities suffered by women is the standard gynaecological examination.

In truth, there is no other logical way of doing it apart from lying on a couch, feet in stirrups and innards on full display to the doctor, the nurse and any passing medical student in search of somewhere dark and hidden to dispose of their chewing gum.

That is no comfort, however, when you're lying there, vulnerable and embarrassed, watching the examiner pull on his or her rubber gloves. Out comes the speculum – looking like a medieval instrument of torture – and the lubricating gel. Finally, the magic word: relax.

Just the thought makes your hair stand on end. And yet, and yet... women have not always been coy about their bodies. In this chapter, we'll see that our forebears were utterly practical in their pursuit of workable contraception and were only too happy to explore their bodies so they could insert barrier methods with confidence.

With advanced civilization and religion came modesty and a series of taboos that still have currency. We stopped being pragmatic and became dramatic.

In recent times, thanks to comediennes, such as Joan Rivers, making jokes about their private parts and shows such as The Vagina Monologues, the mystique surrounding that no-man's-land between a woman's legs is being eroded. Nonetheless, even as we're joining in the laughter, most of us remain ignorant about how things work down there – or even how they look.

Today, barrier methods have a much lower take-up than other forms of contraception. Maybe this chapter will blow away the cobwebs.

Fruit Rinds and Herbal Plugs

Long before contraception was given a name and a practical scientific framework, women were shoving objects into their vaginas with the express intention of stopping sperm in its tracks. More than two centuries ago, Giovanni Giacomo Casanova (1725–98) famously fashioned the Western precursor of the cap by fitting his women with squeezed lemon halves, into which he blasted his seed.

This clearly isn't as outlandish an idea as it first appears. Casanova, despite his myriad exploits, never found himself facing a paternity suit thanks to his lemon aids. And if you think about the thickness and strength of the lemon rind, and the smooth waxiness of its skin, it's infinitely preferable to some of the other options that were on offer.

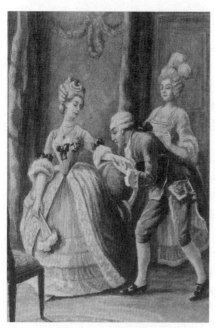

The legendary lover Casanova was an innovator. As well as being one of the most celebrated users of the linen condom, he also invented his own barrier method with lemons.

Indeed, it may well have been his excellent pre-prep that got the Lothario across bedroom thresholds in the first place, as he was known across Europe as a cad, having first distinguished himself in the art of love while studying for the priesthood. In pen portraits, one is not struck by the Latin lover's good looks, but women apparently fell into his arms with their legs wide open.

Casanova turned his exploits into good, bawdy reading, and it is through his Mémoires that we become aware of his expertise at self-protection. That said, the Italian stallion was not the first to think of a cap-like device as a method of birth control.

The principle behind lemon logic was common currency across the world.

In Africa, women devised all sorts of devices to prevent sperm reaching the entrance to the cervix. Using the same technique as that employed by Casanova, they scooped out the inside of seed pods and placed these inside the vagina.

In Greece, where the myth of Persephone and the pomegranate seeds was common currency, women used pomegranate shells in the same way – scooping out the innards and pushing them up against the entrance to the cervix. This was indeed a double protection, as the seeds of the fruit contain a type of oestrogen and therefore do have some contraceptive properties of their own.

But not all the devices were cap-shaped. Some Africans used mixtures of grass and roots, which they rolled into balls and inserted into their vaginas to act as barriers to the seepage of sperm, and to disable movement. In Japan and other parts of the Orient, they inserted mounds of seaweed, moss and bamboo.

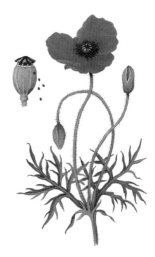

Balls of opium were also used. Opium comes from the seed of the *papaver somniferum* poppy and is famed for reducing pain and inducing a general feeling of soporific well-being. The painkiller morphine is an opiate, as are codeine and the class-A drug, heroin. Opium is highly addictive at all stages of processing.

Three thousand years ago, the ancient Sumerians – they of the first known civilization in Mesopotamia, what is now modern Iraq – called it the joy plant. The Sumerians enjoyed a highly sophisticated lifestyle – they installed irrigation systems to water the land, enjoyed the arts and created beautiful pottery. They invented cuneiform – the earliest form of writing in man's history.

The poppy is commonly associated with heroin in modern society, but in times past unrefined opium was used to block sperm.

They also passed opium along all major trading routes so that it soon started sprouting up all over the place. One can only imagine the after-effects of lovemaking when opium was used as a barrier and, presumably, absorbed by the tip of the penis and the soft tissue inside the vagina.

Wax and Paper Plugs

Further along the timeline, the Germans placed discs of beeswax across the cervix. Because it does not absorb liquid, it's not surprising that beeswax was considered suitable as a barrier method. The body does, however, warm wax, and we have seen how it was used to affix the wishbone pessary, a form of IUD, within the cervix (see page 55). How effective wax was on its own is not recorded.

Beeswax is an amazing substance secreted in the abdominal glands of the honey-bee, and it has been used in the making of candles for hundreds of years because it burns slowly and smells sweet. More recently, we've seen it as an ingredient in skin creams and other cosmetics.

The Persians and Syrians also used beeswax, although not as an aid to contraception. Instead, they coated the bodies of revered public figures in it before burial. After the execution of King Louis XVI and his queen, Marie Antoinette, in 1793, the famous maker of effigies, one Madame Tussaud, used beeswax to make their death masks.

In Asia, female sex workers who needed to prevent pregnancy hit upon the idea of inserting paper discs covered in oil into the vagina, presumably because sperm could not penetrate a barrier of greater viscosity. Indeed, oil as a preventive was recommended well into the twentieth century. It has been seen, historically, as benign.

In the ninth century, a Persian doctor daubed ginger water onto paper, which he fashioned into a tampon-like device and inserted into female patients before intercourse. Anyone who has drunk ginger tea knows how it can burn the tissues of the throat, so goodness knows what sensations this method caused in the vagina, or if there is any evidence that ginger burned off sperm.

Sponges and Wooden Plugs

The Persian invention mirrored that of the ancient Hebrews, who effectively made the first tampons using natural sea sponge. Sea sponge is the prototype of the modern synthetic contraceptive sponge, carrying spermicide neatly into the vagina and working in tandem with vaginal secretions to deter and destabilize any intruders. In biblical times, Jewish women soaked them in vinegar and inserted them into their vaginas, attaching a small cord for ease of removal.

The method is mentioned in the Holy Book of the Jews, the Talmud. Divers in times past risked their lives to swim as much as 100 feet (30m) under water while holding their breath to bring sea sponge to the surface.

Sponge is a living organism surviving on plankton, so we have no idea how much damage was done to natural resources at that time. Once retrieved, the dark membranes of the sponge were removed, leaving just the breathing holes and the soft yellow skeleton – very much like the larger bath sponges that we can now buy in most upmarket chemists. Sponge is retrieved in environmentally efficient ways today to promote regeneration.

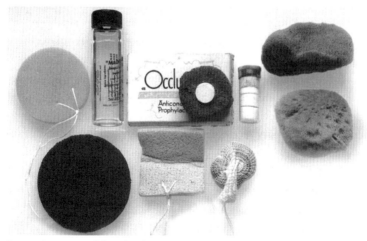

Sponge in its natural form has been used since ancient times as both a barrier to sperm and as a dispenser of spermicide.

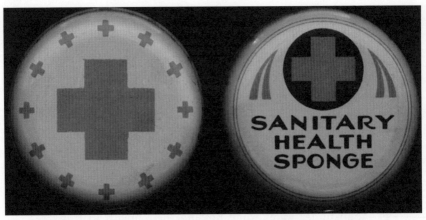

As contraception was frowned upon for religious reasons, methods were often disguised as sanitary ware, as with these spermicidal sponges, which were sold in tins. Menstruating women also used sponges before the tampon was invented.

French women used sponges dipped in brandy as a barrier method in the seventeenth century. And a little further along the timeline, American women used sponges secured inside nets. When immersed in antiseptic, the sponges expanded. The net acted as a container, making the sponges neater and easier to insert. In the early twentieth century, half a dozen sponges cost US$1.25 and a dozen cost US$2, making them too expensive for the casual user.

The sponges were referred to as 'sanitary sponges', thus linking them to menstruation rather than to contraception, which would have gone against the moral grain of those times. They were sold in little tins.

Menstrual sea sponges are available even today. One natural brand called Sea Pearls invites customers to sew a piece of dental floss to their sponges for easy retrieval. If used properly, sponges can last up to a year and are kinder to the vagina than hard tampons, but it does mean that they have to be cleaned and cared for.

But not all barrier methods are kind or even logical, which isn't to say they don't work... German farming families who emigrated to America in the early nineteenth century were found to have smaller families because German midwives placed a little wooden block in front of the patient's cervix.

In rigidly moral Victorian England, women were effectively punished for seeking out barrier methods by being fitted out with carved wooden wedges, which had octagonal sides for ease of insertion and were only dispensed to those who were married. Whether these wooden stops acted as a deterrent to sperm or as a deterrent to sexual intercourse altogether is unclear. These implements were later described as 'instruments of torture'.

Along the same lines, the Maoris had a ritual where stones were placed inside a woman's vagina in the hope that they would make her as sterile as the rocks from which they came. Fortunately, the women were spared the pain of keeping them in place during intercourse.

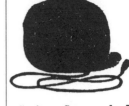

Each in sterile metal box

Sanitary Sponges for Ladies

The above picture is the exact size of one of our soft silk netted sponges when perfectly dry. They are enclosed in a silk netting. When moistened it expands about one-half more than shown. These are extensively used by ladies—when immersed in a good antiseptic and inserted well up into the vagina the passage is kept germ free. Full grown Turkey sponges as fine in texture as velvet.

— Prices —
½ dozen — $1.25
1 dozen — $2.00

— Post Paid —

The sponge is an enduring birth-control favourite, available even now but costing substantially more than US$1.25 for six as they did in the early twentieth century.

Caps and Diaphragms

Before we move on with this history, let's stop for a moment and look at the difference between the cervical cap and the diaphragm, because it starts to matter from the late nineteenth century onwards. I have used the word 'cap' as a generic term for all barrier contraception in this chapter, and will continue to do so. But while the devices are similar in both appearance and application, they are not the same.

To bring it down to lowest common denominator, the differences are more about preference and fitting than anything else. Both are made of latex rubber and can be shaped either like deep prayer caps or large thimbles. However, the cap has a thick folded lip that secures it at the entrance to the cervix, while the diaphragm rests in a

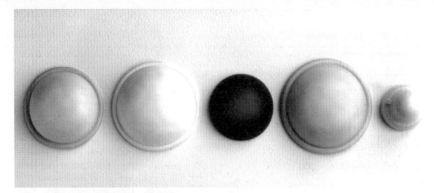

The cap is available in a variety of different sizes, as women are just as individual on the inside as they are on the outside. A thick folded rubber lip distinguishes the cap from the very similar diaphragm.

different manner having, instead of a lip, an adjustable metal rim that secures off the cervix.

With both, there will have to be a moment when you lie back and think of England or America or Australia – or even the Milky Way – and let the nurse or doctor root around to decide which is best for you and in what form. The diaphragm is more adaptable to individual physiology because, as with penises, vaginas come in all shapes and sizes. If you ask your friends they'll no doubt come up with all manner of variations: retroverted wombs, cystoceles, prolapsed wombs and so on, all of which make a difference to the fit of a cap or diaphragm, as does the sizing of a vagina.

Both the diaphragm and the cap require spermicide to be fully effective, and a woman needs to be comfortable with her own body to fit either correctly. Choosing between them is a bit like deciding whether to have a mixed or progesterone-only pill or whether to have a plastic or copper IUD. Whichever is chosen, the principle behind the method remains the same.

It was while she was proselytizing on behalf of the diaphragm that Margaret Sanger was imprisoned in 1916, but we'll come to that period of history shortly, after we've cantered through the leaps of inventiveness that helped turn the principle of the lemon and the seedpod into a mass-produced contraceptive.

The Mensinga Diaphragm became available in the late nineteenth-century and had a major influence on the birth-control movement of the next century.

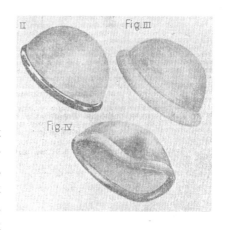

The Cap's Historical Roots

It was a German gynaecologist who came up with the first prototype of the modern cap. In 1838, Friedrich Wilde fashioned what he called 'pessaries' out of rubber, using special moulds to suit individual patients. A quarter of a century later, the American gynaecologist E. B. Foote described a cap-type barrier method in one of his pamphlets. But it was in the 1880s that the method became fully public, thanks to another German gynaecologist called Haase.

Because contraception was still a contentious area, Haase, who had invented a sophisticated diaphragm with a spring-loaded rim, chose not to draw attention to himself. Using the pen name Wilhelm P. J. Mensinga, he wrote a paper introducing what would become known as the Mensinga Diaphragm. It not only brought controversy but also changed the issues surrounding birth control forever.

Because the device was so simple and successful, it was seized

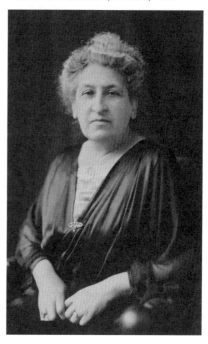

Aletta Jacobs was an extraordinary woman and birth-control pioneer, establishing the world's first family-planning clinic in Amsterdam, Holland in 1878.

upon by Aletta Jacobs, a young Jewish woman who opened the world's first family-planning clinic in Amsterdam. Jacobs, who was also the first woman to qualify as a doctor in the Netherlands, constantly challenged the taboos surrounding birth control.

Jacobs started dispensing the diaphragm from her offices in 1882, so perhaps this is where the term *Dutch cap* originated. Much later, it came to the notice of the woman who would change contraceptive history forever by initiating work on the Pill (see pages 112–14), Margaret Sanger.

Margaret Sanger

Born in 1879 (just three years before Jacobs began dispensing the cap), Margaret Sanger blasted her way onto the contraception map in 1914, with the publication of her pamphlet, *Family Limitation*. In it she listed all manner of douches and sponge applications as workable birth control. But during a trip to Holland in 1915, when she went to visit Jacobs, she learnt about the Mensinga Diaphragm and, as a result, turned a large part of her energies to its importation.

There was only one problem: she was breaking a series of notorious rulings called the Comstock Laws, introduced in 1873 and named after the politician who devised them. Under Comstock, it was illegal to send obscene material through the post, and under the general heading of obscene materials came contraception.

Just by talking about the diaphragm, Sanger was taking on the system and she soon found herself jailed for singing the praises of the device. Incarceration didn't stop her; instead she reportedly used her month in prison to teach fellow inmates how to use the diaphragm. One can just imagine her discussing the merits of barrier contraception over an hour's free association at lunchtime.

On her release, Sanger, through the auspices of the Birth Control Clinical Research Bureau (BCCRB), an organization she had set up for self-evident reasons, faced a new and bigger hurdle. The Comstock Laws stated that no contraceptive device could be either

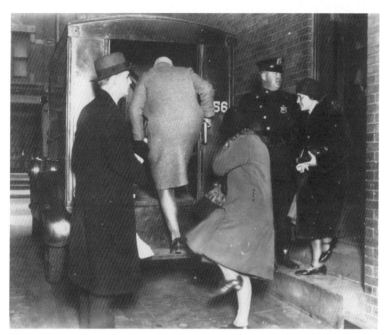

The arrest of Margaret Sanger and her helpers in 1917 for praising the contraceptive merits of the diaphragm focused attention on the iniquities of a system that denied women basic rights over their bodies.

transported or mailed around the United States, thus effectively stopping dispersal of birth control around the federation.

Sanger's second husband, Noah Slee, owned a huge oil company called 3-in-One. Risking everything, he allowed his wife to have diaphragms from abroad packaged in boxes bearing his company logo and imported to the United States, where they were prescribed through the auspices of the BCCRB. At one point, when it became difficult to import the spermicidal gel that went with the diaphragm, he got the recipe and manufactured it himself.

There was a turning point in 1936 when Sanger was taken to court after she was caught in the act of sending a package of 120 Japanese diaphragms to a doctor in New York. The Comstock Laws had by then been thrown out in many cities, including the Big Apple. In an historic judgement, US vs One Package, Sanger got off. It was a

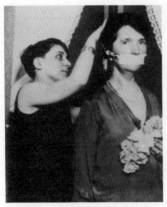

Margaret Sanger spent her life putting her liberty and her reputation at stake for the sake of women's rights. She demanded that birth control be available to the masses and went on to pioneer and help finance the development of the contraceptive pill (see pages 112–47).

decision that undermined and ultimately saw the end of the Comstock Laws.

Later, Sanger would seek a more user-friendly and less expensive alternative to the cap; one that didn't require intimate examination and measuring by doctors, or the associated medical bills. But at that point in the development of birth control, the diaphragm was crucial.

The Pros and Cons of the Cap

Since then, the cap has evolved and it continues to be used across the world. One friend of mine, who has a private gynaecologist in Harley Street, has always sworn by the honey cap, which is a mesh cap impregnated with beeswax, much like the German forerunners. Other variations exist, including a disposable cap that can be worn internally for three days before being thrown away.

That said, with the introduction of non-invasive methods, women are less eager to be instructed on the insertion of foreign objects into the birth canal, particularly when these objects later have to be removed in a wet and squidgy state.

And yet it is the one method that's completely natural. The Pill is easy to take, but it changes our body chemistry and is also easy to forget. The coil requires no conscious thought after the bleeding problems associated with the initial insertion, but it is, nonetheless, an intruder in our bodies. But the cap, the diaphragm and the sponge are the closest you can get to natural contraception without using ovulation charts and willpower. They are the flying squad of birth control, setting up observation posts and throwing down a

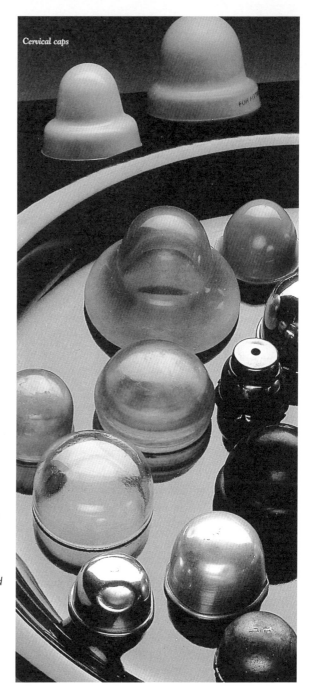

Cervical caps

The cap and diaphragm are similar in application, but the diaphragm has a spring-loaded rim. Both methods are used in conjunction with spermicide and must be left in the vagina for up to eight hours after sexual intercourse.

roadblock when the riff-raff threaten to enter town. Why then do we find them so deeply unsexy?

The main reason is probably that a woman needs to anticipate sex to use the cap or be willing to leap out of bed and insert a piece of curiously moulded latex into her vagina when it becomes clear that intercourse is on the agenda. More seriously, she has to leave the cap inside her for at least eight hours after sex, which could be uncomfortable, filled as she is with both sperm and spermicide.

Spermicides and Modern-day Sponges

Spermicides are nothing new. Spermicide is just a horrible scientific word that means 'potion with sperm-killing properties'. In this book we have looked at many potions that women have used over the millennia, from pessaries steeped in honey to the olive-oil-steeped paper discs.

Modern potions may not be as romantic, but the gels and chemicals we turn out today do eliminate the risk of the formulae being botched. There is even contraceptive film, which comes in little squares that dissolve inside the vagina.

The key ingredient in modern spermicide is Nonoxynol-9, which is used with caps and coated onto condoms. Nonoxynol-9 is a regular ingredient in products as diverse as baby wipes and detergent, but recent reports suggest it can increase susceptibility to HIV when used regularly by women who are already at high risk. For the average woman, however, it's the icing on the birth-control cake.

Unlike caps, contraceptive sponges come impregnated with spermicide (much like the Talmudic version of the sponge soaked in vinegar – see page 63). As a result, the idea of inserting one is marginally less anxiety-filled than dealing with a cap. I do recall, however, a colleague who had trouble retrieving such a sponge from her vagina and was too embarrassed to seek medical help. Thankfully, it later emerged under its own steam, but these situations are best avoided as the side effect of toxic-shock syndrome is not unheard of.

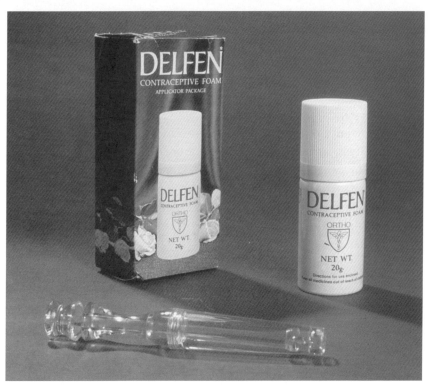

The main ingredient in spermicide is the chemical Nonoxynol-9. Spermicides come in pessary, cream and foam formats, and must be used with caps or diaphragms.

The sponge she used was one that came onto the American market in 1983. It was widely touted in the United Kingdom, too, and soon became popular, but in the mid-1990s, the manufacturers stopped production because of various new laws that pushed the price beyond the pockets of most consumers. It is said that new forms of sponge will soon be on the market, and given their soft flexibility, it's possible that many cap users will prefer them.

A new variation on the cap is the Lea Contraceptive, which looks a bit like a doorbell and knocker, all in one, and doesn't have to be fitted right up against the cervix. Made from silicone, it sucks itself into place and can be inserted up to eight hours before intercourse. Like its peers in the field, it requires the use of a spermicide and must be washed with soap and water after use. There is also the

Femcap, which is more like a sailor's hat and is held in place by its brim.

In ancient times, there were no choices and insertion was often the only way. These days, there is a choice. The inserted device tends to be the option of the woman in a steady relationship who is relaxed and comfortable with her partner; a woman who is not phased by her sexuality or anatomy and for whom a break in the proceedings, if necessary, will not cause a confidence failure.

But it's also a fantastic back-up to have in your handbag in readiness for the unexpected, and remains the one method that doesn't play with the body's functions or require an act of willpower. Cap that, as they say.

Marie Stopes
and the Social Campaign for Birth Control

History and Her-story

One of the most uplifting elements of researching this book was finding out about the women who made birth control possible: women who put their reputations on the line and often lost them as a consequence.

School history books necessarily concentrate on the biggest battles of previous centuries. We all know that the assassination of Archduke Ferdinand of Austria in 1914 precipitated the First World War, in which millions of young men lost their lives.

We are taught about the extraordinary Pankhurst family, Emily, Sylvia and Christabel, who handcuffed themselves to the gates of Buckingham Palace to demand the vote for women.

What we're rarely told is that in the middle of all this turmoil was a group of individuals who were ahead of the game, opening out the debate about women's rights to birth control and, through birth control, self determination.

At a time when more women died through childbirth and related causes than anything else, it was an issue of burgeoning importance. And it was one that was first taken up by socialist thinkers in the nineteenth century.

This is their story, led by the crusader Marie Stopes, who changed the outlook in Britain and influenced global thinking forever.

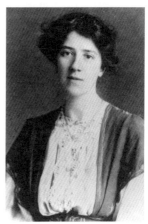

Marie Stopes (1880–1958) campaigned determinedly for birth control against fervent opposition until the medical profession and the general public began to take notice.

Social and Historical Background

In this age of easy come, easy go, we often forget those women and men who put their social and professional reputations on the line to suggest that there was more to sex than making babies: that women had a right to choose between pleasure and pregnancy and that one need not lead to the other.

Like the suffragettes of the early twentieth century, who chained themselves to railings to force the issue on women's voting rights, the early campaigners for accessible contraception had to brave social opprobrium, theological whiteout and patriarchal condemnation. Worse still, like the suffragettes, they also risked imprisonment.

In 1826, the celebrated nineteenth-century activist Richard Carlile (1790–1843) wrote *Every Woman's Book*, which argued for female sexual emancipation through birth control. Despite the uproar that followed, he escaped jail for this perceived social outrage (although he was later imprisoned for other outpourings). Those who supported his views, however, weren't that lucky.

In 1877, Annie Besant and Charles Bradlaugh – members of the free-thinkers movement and acolytes of Carlile – were each sentenced to six months in prison for publishing a book by Charles Knowlton called *The Fruits of Philosophy*, in which the American physician explored the arguments around birth control.

Subtitled 'The Private Companion of Young Married People', *The Fruits of Philosophy* was the first American book of its kind. Originally published in miniature in 1832, it caused Knowlton himself to be imprisoned in his home state of Massachusetts. Besant and Bradlaugh updated the book before publication, and discovered that the British judiciary was no less judgmental than its American counterpart. The judge branded it likely 'to deprave or corrupt those whose minds are open to immoral influences.'

The immorality to which the judge referred was the free-thinkers' challenge to the premise that: 'nice girls don't'. Birth control demeaned the Christian ethic – and so the Establishment ethic – that sex is for procreation, not recreation. It also undermined the tradition of female compliance within a male social order where women were primarily mothers.

In Victorian England, any woman requiring protection was, by implication, looking to indulge in unseemly and ungodly bestial urges outside wedlock. For men, of course, it was a different story and condom shops existed openly in Mayfair, London (see pages 97–99) with proprietors vying for each other's trade. But the condom, it must be remembered, was less about birth control than protection from venereal disease.

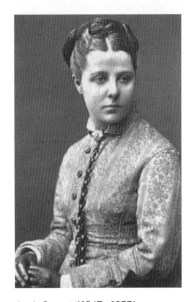

Annie Besant (1847–1933) was a vociferous campaigner for women's rights, and was prosecuted for publishing a book on birth control.

It was only after their case went to appeal that Besant and Bradlaugh escaped imprisonment. But it would take major political upheaval across the whole of Europe for all the various strands in the campaign – the political, the medical and the practical – to come to a point where there could be some form of synthesis. That upheaval came nearly forty years after Besant and Bradlaugh, who later left England to set up shop in India, put their liberty on the line. It came in the form of the First World War (1914–18).

Between 1914 and 1918, over eight million European men, including more than 900,000 young Britons lost their lives. Over two million returned home injured. Simultaneously, there was a communist revolution in the country with the greatest number of soldiers and the greatest number of casualties: Russia.

The whole political map of Europe was changing. Empires were lost and land redistributed. Some regimes were brought low, others were re-energized. Inevitably, as war raged and old ideals were demonized, dismantled or re-assessed, women took on more public roles and gained a stronger voice in the process. One result was that women over the age of thirty were given the vote: but it was hardly enough; they wanted control over their bodies and their fertility too. After all, it had held them back for far too long.

Marie Stopes

In Britain, the most important name to emerge from that consensus was that of Marie Charlotte Carmichael Stopes (1880–1958), and her conversion to the cause started, appropriately enough, in the bedroom. In 1911, Marie Stopes had embarked upon a sexless marriage with a fellow scientist. She knew what was happening – or, rather, not happening – in the bedroom was not ideal, but it wasn't until she'd pored through medical books that she identified her husband's problem as impotence. The marriage was instantly dissolved and as a result her views were changed forever.

On the back of her miserable experience, she wrote a frank and highly controversial book called *Married Love*, exhorting sexual pleasure within marriage for pleasure itself, not just the making of babies: 'In my own marriage I paid such a terrible price for sex-ignorance that I feel that knowledge gained at such a cost should be placed at the service of humanity', Stopes wrote in the foreword to the book. 'I hope it may save... years of heartache and blind questioning in the dark.'

You couldn't make it up: a middle-class English woman, who was still, ostensibly, a virgin, discussing the joys of sex and suggesting that there were two reasons for intercourse – procreation and/or pure pleasure. This was revolutionary at a time when women were still covered from top to toe in order to denote and protect their modesty.

The book was an instant hit and was reprinted within weeks. At this point, Marie Stopes capitalized on the success of *Married Love* with a book that re-focused her ambitions and changed the face of birth control in Britain forever. She decided to write about contraception.

Comically, she had to ask the American birth-control campaigner, Margaret Sanger, what methods were available as she had never had

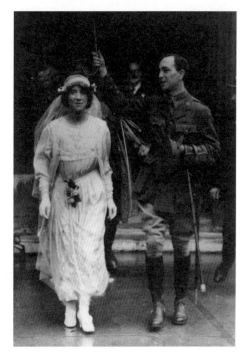

In her second marriage to publisher Humphrey Verdon-Roe in 1918, Marie Stopes finally discovered married love for herself.

a reason to use them. A week later, Sanger turned up at a dinner party with a French pessary in her handbag ('Have a feel of this, dear...') and Stopes's first lesson took place.

In 1917, hot on the heels of her first book, Marie Stopes wrote *Wise Parenthood*. The text took primacy away from the orgasm and placed it, rather more sensibly given her perilous social position, on pacing the rate at which children were being produced. On the back of this, her publisher, Humphrey Verdon-Roe, made a proposal of marriage to Stopes and, having accepted, she discovered the joys of both married love and wise parenthood for herself.

From then on she was unstoppable. In 1921, she defiantly opened the first Marie Stopes birth-control clinic in north London. On the wall of the clinic they put up a declaration that read:

This, the first Birth Control Clinic in the British Empire, was opened on the 17 March 1921, by Humphrey Verdon Roe and his wife Marie Carmichael Stopes, in order to show by actual example what might be done for mothers and their children with no great difficulty, and what should be done all over the world when once the idea takes root in the public mind that motherhood should be voluntary and guided by the best scientific knowledge available.

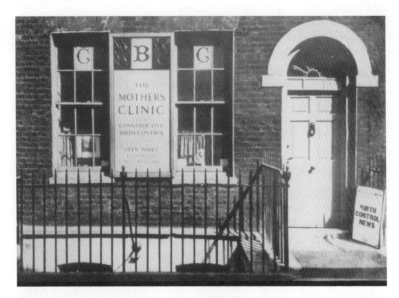

Marie Stopes's first birth-control clinic opened in Holloway, North London in 1921, the first clinic in what is now a worldwide organization promoting birth control and sex education. Below, Marie Stopes and a nurse at the clinic dispense birth-control advice to a couple seeking to plan their family rather than leave it to chance.

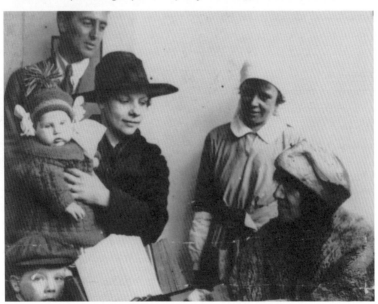

The clinic is free to all, and is supported entirely by the two founders. Those who have benefited by its help are asked to hand on a knowledge of its existence to others and help to create a public opinion which will force the Ministry of Health to include a similar service in Ante-Natal and Welfare Centres already supported by the Government in every district.

The Intelligentsia's Support for Contraception

The clinic was an instant success despite the fact that a hostile climate prevailed. Just two years later, the socialist campaigners Guy Aldred and Rose Witcop were imprisoned for printing Margaret Sanger's arguments in favour of birth control.

But attitudes, while challenged, were not entirely altered. Marie Stopes continued to be reviled by the Establishment, and she was frequently attacked by members of the Catholic Church. One priest wrote: 'It appears to me that a pagan might have written as you do. I had hopes no women would write such books.' Stopes viewed the holy Romans as 'the chief source of evil', but husbands the country over were siding with the clergy as she continued a crusade to, as they saw it, corrupt their wives.

Meanwhile, Aldred and Witcop were behind bars and the intelligentsia, led by Bertrand Russell's wife Dora Black and the economist John Maynard Keynes, were busily fund-raising to buy their freedom. Keynes's economic frameworks would later form the blueprint of Thatcherite thinking, but at that point he was interested in the deregulation of bedroom behaviour.

Keynes was part of a progressive campaign feeding arguments for birth control into the horse's mouth in the hope that by

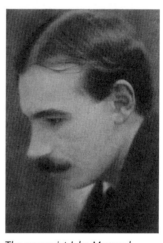

The economist John Maynard Keynes (1883–1946), famed in modern times for his 'trickle-down theory' of economics, added his voice to the growing demand for accessible contraception.

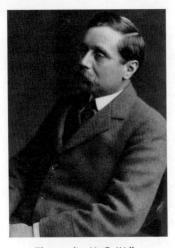

The novelist H. G. Wells was an acclaimed socialist. Rights for women in both the bedroom and the boardroom were fundamental to his philosophy.

the time they trickled down and came out at the other end, enough change would have been implemented to improve the lot of women at grassroots level.

Indeed, deregulation of *coitus* was an issue that excited all progressive intellectuals at that time, including members of the celebrated Bloomsbury Group, who were swinging in all directions behind closed doors. So, it seems, the right for women not to have children went arm in arm with all and any feminist debate.

Even H. G. Wells (1866–1946) who wrote the classic science-fiction novels *War of the Worlds*, *The Time Machine* and *The Island of Doctor Moreau*, got involved and was one of the founders of the Workers' Birth Control Group. He would soon discover that human inconsistency takes longer to resolve than the problems of a sci-fi dystopia.

Eugenics and its Legacy

The intransigence of the Establishment in dealing with the problem does not mean that sex was a social taboo throughout society. No doubt it was discussed in warm terms at market stalls and in bathhouses. I can imagine the women who frequented these places having a good cackle about the ins and outs, so to speak. But the poor were far more disadvantaged by their fertility than their richer sisters in the shires, who could access diaphragms and sponges and put more informed pressure on their husbands to use rubbers.

However, there was a darker side of the original thinking behind birth control. Both Stopes and Sanger were, like all the big thinkers of that time, interested in the eugenics (meaning 'good genes') movement, but this would ultimately come unstuck when taken to its rational extreme by the ugly outrage of Hitler's Germany and the Holocaust.

The birth-control campaigners were at a very different point on the same curve. To put their thinking into context, this was a time when the poor were having huge families and there were no state benefits to support the children. As a result, many were sickly or died, as, often, did their mothers.

Countless women perished in back-street abortions or from taking poisonous herbal remedies to terminate a pregnancy.

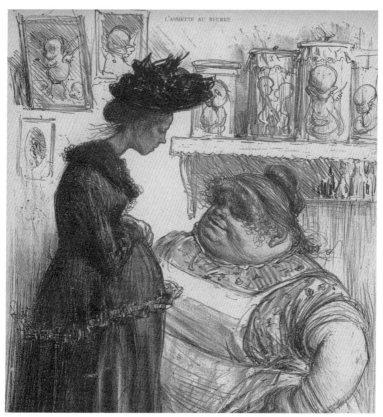

This poignant nineteenth-century cartoon sums up the power of the back-street abortionists and the vulnerability of women who had no control over their own or their husband's fertility. At this point in history, more women were dying from botched abortions than in childbirth.

Indeed, at one point more women were dying as result of abortion than childbirth.

Discouraging poor women from having too many babies was seen as a legitimate reason for backing birth control and, on the surface, looked to have a benign intent. But that intent was underpinned by some deeply unpleasant arguments.

Sanger once said that contraception would allow us 'to create a race of thoroughbreds'. More bizarrely, Stopes raged when her son married a woman who wore glasses because she believed that their resulting children would cause degeneration in the family's genetic legacy.

That intellectual obsession with genetics and social engineering has since been hijacked by the anti-abortion movement to discredit the motivation of organizations dispensing contraception and abortion. And while eugenics and its supporting movements have been entirely discredited, there is, superficially at least, little that separates the underlying principles of the early birth-control lobby from today's arguments.

In the constant debate about under-age sex and the increase in single mothers, it's not society belles or celebrities, such as Tamara Beckwith and Liz Hurley, that we berate for accidentally getting pregnant, it's the young women on sink estates with five children all by different fathers.

In other words, the anxiety about access to birth control is still centred on the poor and the less educated. The aim is to get members of this social group to take responsibility for both their sexual behaviour and its consequences in order to lessen the burden of their welfare on the State. The arguments in favour of contraceptive control are played out against a background of statistics that show that the progeny of the underachievers themselves underachieve, become criminalized, are often without known fathers, and are frequently welfare-dependent.

What is clear is that, while we may have changed the *reasoning* behind the exhortation for the use of birth control, we have not changed the reason. All women have benefited from the free availability of contraception, but it's still the poor who are targeted in any campaign.

What we must not forget, however, are the huge numbers of women that died in childbirth or from abortions in the early twentieth century. Infant mortality was also high due to poor housing and poverty. There was good reason to target those on the bottom rung. Nonetheless, Hitler's decision to take eugenic thinking to its murderous and terrible extreme exposed the danger of espousing a hierarchical philosophy.

For all this, Marie Stopes, whatever her motivation, changed the odds for poor and rich alike. *Married Love*, which sowed the seeds for all the theories that would follow, is considered to be one of the most influential books of the twentieth century.

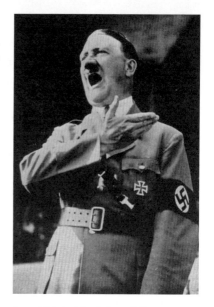

Eugenicist doctrine informed the birth-control movement in its early days, but when Adolf Hitler (1889–1945) and Nazi Germany took such thinking to its ultimate extreme, the leading birth-control advocates immediately distanced themselves from it.

Jacobs, Stopes and Sanger

Stopes was not, of course, the only European agitating for change. Indeed, in some ways, she was way behind the rest, because freer attitudes towards sexuality were then, and still are, prevalent in other parts of Europe.

In Amsterdam in 1878, Holland's only female doctor, Aletta Jacobs, had opened a contraceptive clinic (see page 67). Having started out with a clinic teaching Dutch women hygiene and childcare, Jacobs realized there was a need for birth control and came across a spring-loaded diaphragm called the Mensinga Diaphragm (see pages 67–8) which she prescribed from her clinic until her retirement in 1904.

Like her successors, Jacobs was very much influenced by the Malthusian thinking she had encountered in London in the late nineteenth century. The economist T. R. Malthus (1766–1834) postulated that the population rate increases faster than its means of subsistence, and should, therefore, be checked through sexual restraint. Also, like her successors, she encountered hostility to her ideas and actions: 'They accused me of promoting abortion and of leading an immoral life,' she later wrote. But when she confronted her accusers: 'The culprit… would shrug it all off with some remark about contraception being the same as abortion.'

It was hard going, and the truth couldn't have been more different. None of the women who campaigned for, and dispensed, birth control was promiscuous or immoral. Jacobs and Sanger came from solid medical backgrounds, and this bound them together. Stopes was very different, but she came from a middle-class family of high achievers, one of whom, unusually for those times, was her mother.

Stopes's mother was academically brilliant. She pushed her daughter to follow in her footsteps, and Marie won a science scholarship to University College, London in 1901. An effortless student, she got a double first in botany in less than the usual time and by 1905 had completed her PhD. and was lauded as Britain's youngest doctor of science. She came to birth control purely through feminist politics and her own miserable experience of marriage.

What Stopes and Jacobs had in common was that they both went on to campaign in other areas of the female struggle for equality by leaving their established clinics in the hands of others. Sanger battled on alone, campaigning solely for birth control and starting the Planned Parenthood Federation, now an international body advising governments across the world on population control.

It was Sanger who demanded an oral contraceptive for women, found the funding to research it, and died an octogenarian with millions of women the world over thanking her (see pages 112–26).

But we're getting ahead of ourselves, because what's important here are the heroines who pushed the foundation stones of female contraception into place. Without them, the layout of the contraceptive timeline might be very different...

Stopes's influence cannot be overstated. Her books in themselves ensured her immortality, but she also eased the passage for those campaigners who followed in her wake.

The Founding of the Family Planning Association

One such campaigner was Lady Gertrude Denman (1884–1954), a rich and well-connected feminist who was Chairman of the Women's Institutes. She would later form the Women's Land Army that took over the running of two million acres of agricultural land during the Second World War (1939–45).

Denman was very interested in birth control and set up the National Birth Control Council in the 1930s, appointing a married woman with a young son as its first secretary. That woman was Margaret Pyke (1893–1966), and she would soon become the leading light in the field.

In 1939, Pyke cleverly changed the name of the organization to the more user-friendly Family Planning Association (FPA) and started opening advisory clinics around Britain.

Over a twenty-year period, using a softly-softly approach, Pyke pushed back the frontiers even further and in doing so widened women's choices while winning the ear, and eventually the backing, of the Government. But she could only win by *pushing* at the barriers to change, not by hammering them with a battering ram. On that basis, the FPA offered help and advice only to those women who were married and had a 'legitimate' claim to help.

This impasse seriously concerned one of the FPA's younger members. Helen Brook, chair of an FPA in north London, was unhappy that the organization was denying contraceptive advice to the unmarried. It was, by now, the early 1960s. Elvis Presley was swivelling his hips – though they couldn't be shown on

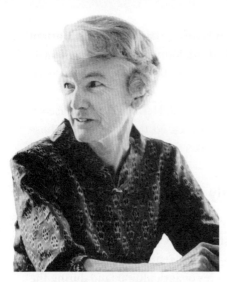

Margaret Pyke (1893–1966) learned to play the political system for her own ends, but it wasn't until after her death that local authorities sanctioned the dispensing of contraceptives.

television – the Pill had just been invented and, appropriately, Bob Dylan was singing 'The times, they are a-changing.' Why, Brook asked, can't we change too?

In the preceding years the FPA had been forced to rethink its strategies on many fronts. They were involved in debates over marital discord, the age of consent, Thalidomide and, from 1963, abortion (see pages 127–42). But the issue of sex outside marriage still seemed to be a bridge too far.

At the 1964 Annual General Meeting of the FPA, the organization's Honorary Secretary, Nancy Raphael, came up with a solution: there should be a separate service dealing with the needs of young people.

Helen Brook took this as her calling; she cut free from the mother ship and opened her own service, The Brook Advisory Service, providing contraception for those women who were old enough to know their own minds and wise enough to protect their bodies. The contraceptive revolution was moving into the final stages of emancipation.

Margaret Pyke died in 1966 when the FPA was still dependent on the kindness of benefactors to survive and when all birth control was privately dispensed. After her death and the 1967 Abortion Act, local authorities were given permission to dispense contraceptive advice legally and help all women, irrespective of marital status.

In 1969, Prince Philip gave the royal seal of approval to the movement by officially opening The Margaret Pyke Centre in London, now the headquarters of the Family Planning Association.

Today, the legacies of Pyke and Brook, like that of Stopes, who died quietly in 1958, are continued through their organizations.

The Legacy of the Pioneers

Stopes later got involved in other feminist issues: she fought to stop education authorities discriminating against married female teachers and she demanded that men and women should be taxed separately – until relatively recently, it was British fathers who had child allowances included in their tax codes, and not the mothers.

She also ran a newspaper called *Birth Control News* until her death. Today, her organization is still run from the original building in central London where she started. Marie Stopes International pursues and compounds a woman's right to choose, from the dispensing of pills, potions and prophylactics to the carrying out of terminations in cases where the former either didn't work or were forgotten in the heat of the moment.

The Family Planning Association came under the auspices of the National Health Service in 1976, when it was decided that contraception should be free of charge and freely available. The Margaret Pyke Memorial Trust, a registered charity, continues with research, education and training separate to the Margaret Pyke Centre and the FPA.

The Brook Advisory Service is a charitable organization that has shortened its name to Brook, and concentrates on helping those under twenty-five with advice and contraception. Lady Helen Brook is still active in the field.

In the space of four generations, we have gone from left-wing campaigners being imprisoned for promoting contraception, to easy availability of the morning-after pill (see page 138)

The achievements of Stopes, Pyke and Brook cannot be over-stated. In 1924, a twenty-seven-year-old woman who was expecting her fourth child wrote this letter to Marie Stopes: 'My children do not have enough to eat… I have got into trouble with the school, because my boy did not go, as I had no boots for him to wear. My mother… says I must stop having children. Do you think it would be best if I leave my husband and go into the workhouse… so we do not have any more?'

This letter was written in the lifetime of our parents and grandparents. On that basis, it is perhaps not surprising that so many older people find it difficult to accept the ease with which birth control is dispensed today – to them, it appears that we have gone from one extreme to the other.

But whatever one's view is on public morality, what cannot be underplayed is the drive, the courage and the indomitable spirit of those women who formed the birth-control movement and liberated their sisters, high and low equally, from the tyranny of unplanned or unwanted pregnancy.

The Condom
Something for the Weekend

Condoms A-Go-Go

There is the old joke about the nun working in the condom factory who believes she's making hats for gnomes. But, as we know, size isn't an issue when talking condoms.

Well, actually, it is: and will, I hope, provide some light relief in this chapter. Not that light relief is hard to come by when discussing this particular form of birth control. More commonly, one is dogged by a need to sober up and take it seriously.

The condom is a method of contraception that naturally ranks among the oldest. After all, the suppression of sperm is the most obvious way to prevent pregnancy.

Given that until relatively recently it was believed that sperm alone – without the necessary ovum – made babies, what's surprising is not that men have devised so many different ways of sheathing their penises over the centuries, but that they didn't make more.

One of the biggest problems, historically, was finding ways of keeping a condom attached to the male tool. All manner of ribbons were used, which must have been rather restrictive. Perhaps the ribbon acted in the same way as today's penis rings – prolonging the act and the pleasure.

Pleasure or pain, the condom's stature remains undiminished as more sophisticated techniques are found to make it more like a second skin than a second coating.

In an era where sexual health is literally a matter of life or death, it is a barrier that cannot be recommended highly enough, even for those already using other forms of contraception.

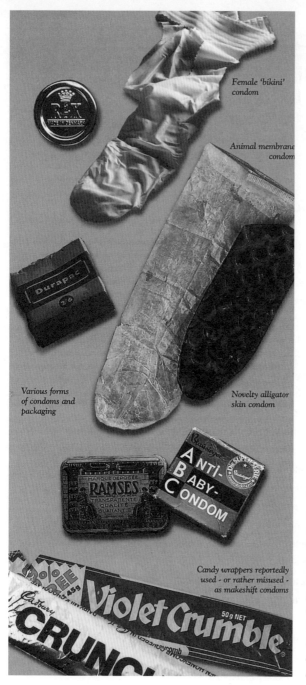

Female 'bikini' condom

Animal membrane condom

Various forms of condoms and packaging

Novelty alligator skin condom

Candy wrappers reportedly used - or rather misused - as makeshift condoms

The principle of the condom predates the modern latex models, but both old and new prophylactics were devised not primarily as methods of birth control but as protective measures for men against venereal disease.

A Name's a Name

In the old days, the usual way for a man to get a condom was to go to the barber's shop where, as his last whiskers were whisked off, the crimper would lean forward and ask knowingly: 'Something for the weekend, Sir?'

Condom is not an ugly word, like diaphragm; or a peculiar notion, like the sponge; or unimaginatively basic, like the Pill; but it does invite euphemism. There is something about the concept, or perhaps its celebration of the Priapic, that is essentially laughable. Not that penis-worship made Casanova laugh: he would ejaculate while prostitutes tried different sizes of homemade condoms on his tool.

During successive modern wars, soldiers (those who were allowed to have condoms, that is, and I'll come to that later) referred to them as 'rubber Johnnies'. In the United States, 'rubber' is the common diminutive. In the United Kingdom a brand name is commonly used as a generic: Durex. But these terms refer directly to the modern condom, which is made of vulcanized tree sap.

Favourite names that predate rubber condoms still persist, including 'French letter' or 'Frenchie'. On the European mainland, conversely, condoms are known as 'English overcoats' or 'raincoats'.

In this book, though, we call a condom a condom. So let's first consider where the name comes from. Every other form of contraception we look at has a line of progression that explains its title. In medical terms, a contraceptive pessary is just that. And you couldn't find a more literal description than the cap. An Intra-uterine Device is precisely what it says. So, whither condom?

The earliest condoms found in Britain were located in the lavatories at Dudley Castle and date back to the English Civil War (1642–9). The story has it that a Colonel Quondam kitted out Royalist soldiers with the rudimentary cover-alls. Given that there is material evidence of condoms being used, this is possible. But was there really a Colonel Quondam?

The sheathing of the willy to stave off unplanned misfortunes ('sheath' being another semantic alternative) became very important in bawdy Restoration times, and an alternative version of the story has it that Condom was the name of a physician in the court of King Charles II. He is credited with fashioning the original sheep's gut version to protect promiscuous willies from the hideous deformities bestowed by the clap during licentious bonking.

However, in my searches I could not find the origin of this claim. That said, the seventeenth century was certainly a busy time in English history. What with the Great Plague, followed quickly by the Great Fire of London and the endless vacillating over religion and politics, it's hardly surprising that the men of the court constantly sought extra-curricular fun and had, therefore, to be protected from themselves.

It's All Greek...

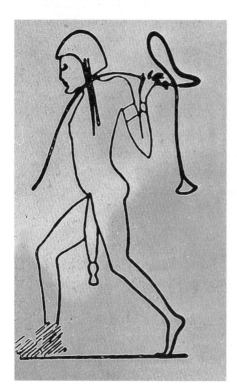

In Greek mythology, King Minos of Crete is variously described as using a fish's bladder or a goat's bladder as a tool of protection for his tool of procreation. It probably protected his partners, too, as he reportedly boasted scorpions and serpents in his semen. For a king born as the result of a rape – that of his mother, Europa, by the god, Zeus – such caution is understandable. But his protective measures didn't stop his wife from giving birth to their son, Theseus.

This earliest known image of a protective sheath dates back some 3,000 years to Ancient Egypt.

The legend of Minos dates back 5,000 years. By 1000 BC, the myth had become a reality, with the ancient Egyptians reportedly wearing linen sheaths as protection, not from unwanted babies but from a disease called Bilharzia, caused by an aquatic worm entering the body through all and any orifices. Sexual protection then was about protection from disease, not from the demands of the Family Court.

There is an illustration supposedly dating back to around 1300 BC of a man with an extremely large condom, complete with teat – the squishy little bit at the end for catching the sperm. Quite how historians have extrapolated that this ancient Egyptian appendage is a prophylactic (a medical term meaning a procedure or tool for the prevention of disease) and not an artist's impression of the willy itself is beyond me, as, to the untrained eye, it could be either. Have a look at the illustration (opposite) and see what you think...

Falloppio and Casanova's English Riding Coats

In the French caves of Combarelles, famous for Paleolithic rock, are drawings of all animal life, including donkeys, cave lions and rhinos. Also among the etchings that remain are drawings dating back to 100 and 200 BC that purportedly show men wearing condoms.

The first written record of the condom, however, comes from Italy: a fact that also lends credibility to the argument that the word condom comes from the Latin condon, meaning 'receptacle'.

It is to the Italian anatomist Gabriello Falloppio that we turn at this point. He is a man whose memory lives on within all of the fairer sex, thanks to his discovery and recording of the Fallopian tubes. A brilliant man, the workings of the human body were his passion.

In 1564, two years after Falloppio died, his book on syphilis, De Morbo Gallico, was published and with it details of condoms he had made from linen and distributed and tested on his male patients. Falloppio's sheaths were dipped in salt and herbs and tied under the foreskin with a ribbon – ouch. What effect this had on performance or blood flow is not recorded, but clearly there must have been some success in pre-

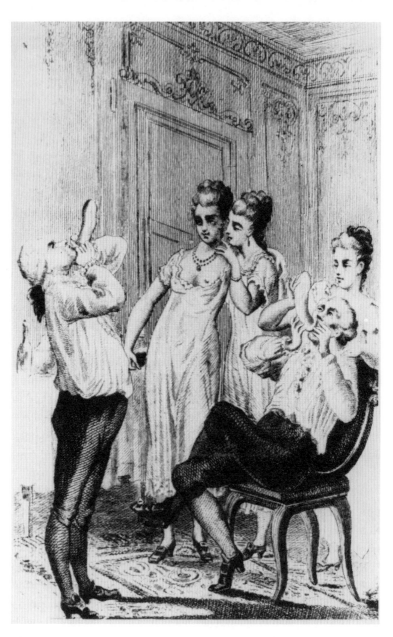

The great Italian lover Casanova blows up a condom in this nineteenth-century drawing. The male contraceptive has long been a point of ridicule and humour.

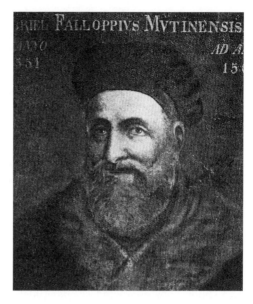

The Italian anatomist Gabriello Falloppio (1523–62) lives on in women. It was he who identified the tubes that carry the female egg from the ovary to the uterus – the Fallopian tubes – and he was prolific in the area of birth control.

venting men from impregnating their partners or catching horrid diseases or the practice would not merit mention.

A couple of hundred years on, Casanova too, was using condoms – his, like those recommended by Falloppio, were made of linen. He called them his 'English Riding Coats'.

Intestines and English Raincoats

But in the battle between linen and innards, it was the innards that won. Over time it became generally accepted that the superior material for fashioning condoms was animal intestine – a thought that elicits horror in the modern man and woman, not just because of the device's provenance, but because of the pungency of animal matter. Better pungent, however, than pregnant.

Smell didn't pose a problem for royalty of that time. They could afford to demand the best, and soon de luxe versions were on offer. Louis XVI had his condoms lined with velvet and silk and delivered by diplomatic bag from London. He called them *capote d'anglais* – English raincoats.

The condom was the new black. In 1724, White Kennett wrote a poem with the following lines:

Hear and attend: In cundum's praise
I sing and thou, O Venus! aid my lays.
By this Machine, secure, the willing Maid
Can taste Love's Joys, nor is she more afraid
Her Swelling Belly should or squalling brat,
Betray the luscious Pastime she had been at.

It was also in the eighteenth century that Mathijs van Mordechay Cohen opened the first dedicated condom shop in Amsterdam.

In London's Mayfair, not far from the notorious Shepherd's Market where even today young women of questionable repute ply their wares, two supposedly respectable ladies, Mrs Phillips and Mrs Perkins, sold all manner of *baudruches* (from the French meaning balloon and animal intestine) and *armour* (associated with the Italian, and English word for protective clothing). From their respective shops, they competed via pamphlets in which each criticized the other's wares.

For the man whose penis activity did not match his earning abilities, there was, apparently, a Miss Jenny who handwashed condoms that had been used by previous owners, and sold them as nearly new.

A recipe for animal-gut protection dating back to 1824 reveals that, even then, condoms were categorized as fine and superfine. What differentiated the former from the latter was that the superfine were double-washed and soaked for a longer time. They were then scented with essences and polished against glass. There was also a superfine double condom which was literally that: one *baudruche* moulded onto another.

Once you'd bought your condom you still needed to soak it before use to make it supple, and in some paintings of the time you can see them hanging on the line to dry.

What we have here is the slow but steady acceptance of across- and under-the-counter contraceptive remedies, whatever the primary reasons for their popularity. But even at this point in history, there wasn't a universal recipe or manufacturing method that could provide condoms in the numbers required.

Then the Industrial Revolution happened and everything changed, including the ready availability of protection.

The Rise of the Rubber

In 1838, the American Charles Goodyear invented a method for vulcanizing India rubber. Vulcanizing effectively means heating the freshly-tapped sap – latex – from the *hevea brasiliensis* tree, with a sulphur mixture. The heating process makes the rubber so elastic it can be cross-linked in microscopic layers, building up an extraordinary tensile strength.

Within five years, the method was patented (though the patent was ignored so often that Goodyear, whose invention revolutionized the manufacturing process, died a poor man), and condoms started to roll off the factory lines. Mass production was under way.

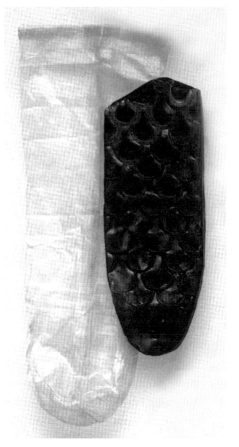

These may look like odd socks found at the bottom of the laundry basket, but these generously cut sheaths are nineteenth-century condoms. The more a gentleman had to spend, the more luxurious the item he could buy.

As ever, the end of one problem merely heralded the beginning of a whole catalogue of new conundrums. Condoms may have been made by the bucket-load, but this didn't mean that Tom, Dick and Harry were queuing round the block to purchase them.

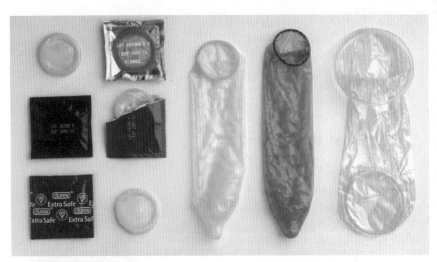

Modern condoms come in different shapes, sizes and textures for personal preference. On the right of the picture is the female condom – the Femidom– which has never reached the same level of popularity as the traditional male version.

In England and America, Victorian values were embraced as the ideal. Society was enlightened when it came to learning and philanthropy, but rigid and hidebound in matters that touched upon public morality. The theologians worried that contraception was not Christian, and that condoning its use would help promulgate arguments for birth control, including handing some choice to women.

War and Social Revolution

It was with the First World War (1914–18) that the condom became accepted common currency. With millions of lonely and vulnerable men out in the trenches, comfort was sought, and there was, inevitably, much use of brothels.

Marie Stopes's first West End clinic in Whitfield Street preferred to encourage women to use female contraceptive techniques rather than rely on male involvement. However, it did make condoms available, and it was the only outlet from which women could acquire them.

SPACING BABIES FOR HEALTH
The Use of Condoms
(Popularly called Sheaths or French Letters).

The fundamental teaching of our President and the Mothers' Clinics has been that contraceptives used by the male are less physiologically right than the best type used by women. The C.B.C. Committee is still strongly of the opinion that where possible the wife should be properly fitted at a Clinic with the contraceptive best for her own use.

Some people are so placed that they cannot visit a Clinic immediately after marriage. Moreover there is no clinically recommended feminine method which can be used by virgin girls, and so brides cannot be reliably fitted until a few weeks of marriage have passed. These, and other factors in our social life sometimes make the use of the condom by the man temporarily advisable.

The commercial trade in condoms is generally profiteering, and often has unpleasant associations. For many years the C.B.C. Society, disliking their use, left patients coming to its Clinics unhelped regarding condoms.

As exposed in the House of Commons Debate recent commercial developments have become so offensive that the C.B.C. Committee, after mature consideration, decided that it would be failing in its duty if it did not make it possible for those needing help to obtain through its irreproachable source reliable and inexpensive condoms.

Every type has been tested most carefully and the C.B.C. now supplies really satisfactory thin condoms or sheaths.

Packets of three for 1/-
(Postage 2½d.)

The C.B.C. Committee considers that these condoms at three for 1/- will solve many of the problems which have unfortunately accumulated round the provision of this type of contraceptive.

Special price to Doctors £1. 18. 0. for a gross Condoms (in packets of 3).

Cash with order.

That didn't stop the God-squadders from sabotaging efforts to maintain the good health of the troops. The American Social Hygiene Association, which believed that venereal disease was the price you paid for the sin of copulating with strange women, objected to the boys of the American Expeditionary Forces being issued with condoms – so they weren't. The soldiers helped to liberate Europe, but Europe enslaved many of them to the ball and chain of sexually transmitted diseases.

The British were more sensible. The high incidence of venereal disease led army chiefs to distribute sheaths that had been treated with antiseptic ointments in the hope of cutting down the problem.

As the war ended, people like Marie Stopes in Britain (see pages 75–90) and Margaret Sanger (see pages 68–70) in America had already got the birth-control bandwagon rolling so that contraception could be discussed publicly.

Interestingly, Stopes, Britain's leading expert, disapproved of the condom. She claimed that semen was a natural stimulant that nourished a woman's body and that the condom was a barrier to a woman's sexual satisfaction. At the time, her arguments were ignored, but it has been proved in the twenty-first century that she was absolutely right: the chemicals in semen induce a feeling of well-being in women.

The Contribution of Durex

Meanwhile, the whole process of latex manufacture was undergoing a sophisticated make-over that would also re-educate men. In London, one L. A. Jackson was forming the London Rubber Company (LRC) in a back room. One of the first things he did was to organize the importation of 'protectives' from Germany, which he distributed through barbers' shops. Hence, 'Something for the weekend?'

In 1929 LRC registered the Durex (Durability, Reliability, Excellence) trademark and, three years later, opened its own factory in Hackney, east London. By 1930, the company was making condoms from liquid latex which provides a much finer mix but has to be

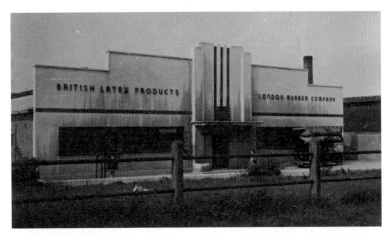

The original London Rubber Company started life in the back room of a barber's shop in 1915, but by the 1930s their success rate was so high and demand was so great that it was operating out of a purpose-built factory, and soon became the founding stone for today's international Durex Empire.

treated very carefully because it's a bit like milk – it goes sour and curdles if it isn't quickly stabilized and compounded.

When, in 1939, the Second World War broke out and condom supplies from Germany dried up, so the LRC increased its output to meet orders to supply the second wave of lovelorn soldiers. This time, even the Americans had got the message and they aggressively promoted the use of precautions with the classic line: 'Put it on before you put it in.' The condom was on the map.

And yet, because there was so much disapproval around the use of contraception, and an implication that anyone seeking it was involved in ungodly acts, not everyone trusted them. Apocryphal stories circulated saying that one in ten condoms was deliberately made faulty to keep the Church happy. Rumours consistently abounded of Catholic factory staff deliberately pricking the rubber so semen would leak.

This line of disinformation was eradicated in 1953 when the LRC introduced electronic testing machines. By 1957, the techniques were so advanced that the first lubricated condom came on the

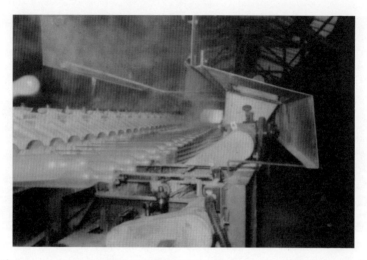

There were rumours that devout Catholics working on the London Rubber Company's production lines were deliberately pricking every tenth condom to encourage them to fail. In the 1960s, however, the introduction of testing batches and the British Standard Kitemark challenged public fears.

market. Every approved condom on the market today has gone through five specific tests. First, they're electronically checked at high voltage to see if the latex breaks down in any way. At that point test batches are removed for more intensive workouts.

Condoms are filled with water and suspended for three minutes to see if there is any fluid leakage. They are then tested for physical strength and durability through artificial ageing. The most surprising test is that for elasticity, which involves blowing up a condom like a balloon (indeed, Marie Stopes likened them to the balloons you could buy at Woolworth's). At this stage they're filled with air. Durex boasts that its condoms only burst at forty litres (which is equivalent to nine gallons of water).

In 1962, the company opened its own family-planning clinic. That year, the National Health Service also started distributing condoms via Margaret Pyke's organization (see pages 87–89).

In 1964, the British Standard Specification for condoms was certified and the little packet of three was given the Kitemark, signifying safety and quality. And yet, this did not lead to a massive demand for condoms among men… because the Pill had come on the market. For the first time, men could be careless without worry, because women were taking on the responsibility.

The Role of the Condom in Birth Control

Elsewhere in the world, however, the condom was heavily promoted. There is a curious story from India about birth-control campaigners wondering why their condom campaign had failed in one particular village. On returning there, they discovered that the demonstrator had used a stick in the ground to demonstrate how a condom should be worn, but had failed to explain that the stick represented the penis. Hence, the village boasted a large number of pregnant women, and sticks in fields wearing condoms.

In Thailand, there was dismay when American condoms, made for men a lot taller and wider, didn't fit too well. It was discovered that even the small difference in size was important when manufacturing prophylactics and changes to manufacturing processes were made accordingly.

Staying with size, the wonderfully named Barbara Seaman, an American writer on birth control, suggested that condom sizes should be classified as Jumbo, Colossal and Super Colossal, 'so that men don't have to ask for small.' Later in the evolutionary chain, companies would rise up selling rubbers especially tailored for the larger man.

But the 1960s, 1970s and early 1980s was a golden time of sexual licence and licentiousness. Who wanted condoms when you could enjoy the sensuality of the real thing, thanks to every second woman being on the Pill? The old fears about venereal disease, which had originally fuelled the condom's popularity, were forgotten as STD (Sexually Transmitted Disease) clinics opened with antibiotics and instant cures for every eventuality from syphilis to trichomoniasis.

Nonetheless, for the very young (who were too embarrassed to seek medical assistance), and the middle-aged (for whom the Pill was

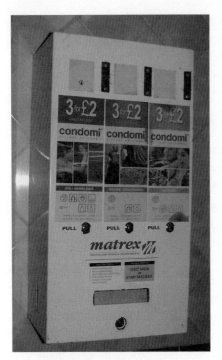

Today, condom machines are ordinary fixtures in pubs and clubs. The first machine appeared in 1967, and they were orginally confined to men's lavatories but can now be found in women's toilets, too.

not advised), and those caught out by an offer of 'lurve' when they were unprepared, the condom machine in men's toilets came to play an important part in the fashioning of modern sexual culture.

To counter the bother associated with the condom – having to stop midway through the warm-up process to inelegantly pull on a rubber – it was given a make-over. Frenchies were produced with ridged sides and strange tentacles wobbling around on the end. They were spewed out in different colours – one for each day of the week: black, pink, blue, green and even striped. And then we had the ultimate – the flavoured condom, 'Chocolate, mint, raspberry or brandy and coke – you take your pick, Doll.'

AIDS and Safe Sex

But when the shadow of AIDS started casting its darkness across the world in the 1980s, the condom came into its own. It had started life as a rank piece of animal tissue tied with a ribbon, but with industrialization it became a back-room Johnny, so to speak – used by those who dare not speak its name for fear of social ostracism and, finally, a cover-all for the dogs of war.

The men of the 1950s had come to rely on it, but by the 1960s they were relying on the women instead. Now there was a red alert on the

Tannoy: 'If you don't use one of these and practise safe sex, you could be writing out not just your own death warrant, but those of the innocents you have loved.'

In the United States, a vociferous gay rights lobby pushed the problem to the top of the political agenda in the early 1980s with the support of celebrities. In the United Kingdom, however, the authorities truned a blind eye until 1985, when its first pro-condom, anti-AIDS campaigns were launched. Initially there was much confusion, because the then British Prime Minister, Margaret Thatcher, wanted the word 'sheath' to be used instead of 'condom'. Unfortunately, few young people knew what a sheath was.

As Elizabeth Taylor and Elton John headed fund-raising galas in the United States, the historic 'iceberg ad' was broadcast on British television and in cinemas, with John Hurt providing a doom-laden commentary. It was made clear that everyone was at risk, not just

The Femidom – a female condom – provides similar protection to the condom, but in order to work it must be fitted over the woman's external genitals as well as within the vagina.

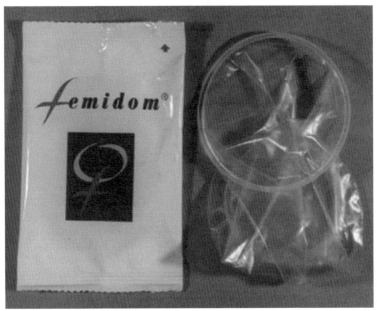

members of the gay community, whom the disease had initially affected most severely. Nonetheless, within the heterosexual community, there was insufficient take-up and women found themselves at risk from HIV.

In 1992, women who didn't trust men to be fastidious in their lovemaking, HIV or no HIV, were given the option of buying a female condom: a polyurethane device that works on the same principle as the male version but does not require an erection to work. Known in the vernacular as a pie-liner, it is fitted over the external genitalia and into the cervix, providing a barrier to sperm in exactly the same way as a male condom, and is advantageous to the man because he is not required to withdraw immediately after ejaculation. Because it is plastic, the Femidom is resistant to both oil- and water-based spermicides and lubricants.

In the twenty-first century, the take-up rate on condoms has improved, but an internet survey held by Durex in 2002, found that large numbers of young people were still prepared to risk unprotected sex with strangers rather than say 'No'. The campaigns continue.

The Ubiquitous Condom

So… we have come full circle. In 1564 Gabriello Falloppio was writing about condoms in the context of syphilis and trying them out on the good men of his parish. In the twenty-first century, although the condom's properties as a contraceptive are long established, it is as much for the protection it offers from HIV and AIDS, herpes and carcinogenic genital warts that we value it as for its birth-control value.

Male or female, pink or black, ridged or plain, normal or large, superfine or gossamer, butterscotch or mint – it will always be the subject of some awkwardness. I remember a story I was told a few

Taking the mystique out of sex: this jovial advert, aimed specifically at school-children, was intended to give the impression that condoms were part of the fun of sex rather than an unwanted interruption.

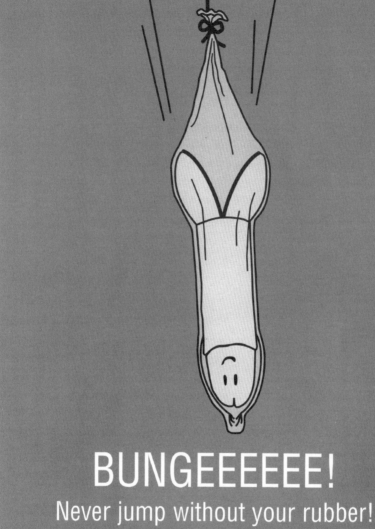

BUNGEEEEEE!

Never jump without your rubber!

EMERGENCY CONTRACEPTION
ABORTION HELP
CONTRACEPTION
HEALTH SCREENING

0845 300 8090
www.mariestopes.org.uk

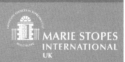

MARIE STOPES
INTERNATIONAL
UK

ONLY CONDOMS HELP PREVENT BOTH STIs AND PREGNANCY

years ago: a friend's mother ran a tobacconist in Kilburn, in north-west London, and one day, a young man came in and sheepishly asked for some condoms. 'Certainly, Sir', she replied. 'Ready rubbed or long cut?' Their shop was next door to the chemist: he hadn't looked and she had misheard. She thought he'd asked for Condor, which was a very fashionable tobacco of the time. His exit was described as 'hasty'.

Nowadays, there's no embarrassment for those teenagers brought up on condom sense. Condoms are displayed alongside toiletries in supermarkets and sold in batches on the internet. Like support stockings, they stay up magically – no ribbons for today's lads – and they're cheap enough not to need rinsing and re-using. Falloppio would be astonished. The rest of us are just plain grateful.

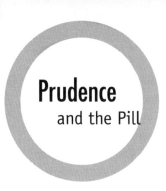

Prudence
and the Pill

The 'It' Contraceptive

Unlike the other chapters in this book, there is no long history that goes with the Pill, as the development of oral contraception has already been covered in earlier pages documenting the use of potions, herbs and other plants that were believed to suppress female fertility.

In the West, the Pill stands alone as a beacon of liberation. However, it does not do so well in cultures where women cannot access clinics on a regular basis to have their blood pressure taken and general health checked before a new batch is dispensed.

More than any other solution, it is a contraceptive that works for the young, and the young, necessarily, are the area of greatest concern – not because they're more promiscuous, but because they're more careless about taking responsibility for themselves.

Pill packets even have the days of the week written on them for ease of reference: they're as close to idiot-proof as one gets, short of an invasive long-term solution.

There is little else to say, other than that the title of this chapter comes from a film of the 1960s – the racily entitled Prudence and the Pill. A comedy starring Deborah Kerr and David Niven, it was the story of a sex-starved husband who, convinced his wife is having an affair, substitutes aspirin for her birth-control pill to see if she gets pregnant.

As they say on kids' programmes after testing a product in dangerous circumstances: this is not an idea we suggest you try at home…

Margaret Sanger and the Pill

Earlier in this book we looked at the movers and shakers of birth control and I mentioned Margaret Sanger in passing, but concentrated on the British side of the equation. This is because the battles being waged by the likes of Marie Stopes were broadly the same across Europe and the United States. Any woman who put her name to the campaign faced imprisonment and social exclusion.

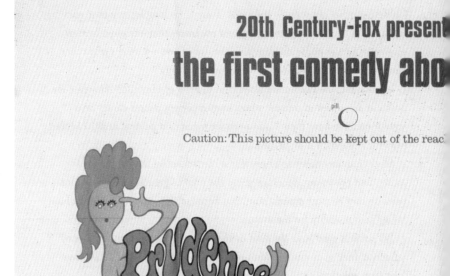

But Margaret Sanger has a peculiar and everlasting claim to fame that puts her in a different league: because it was she who conceived the idea of a birth-control pill – *the* Pill – and then spent her life pursuing it. It is because of her grit and determination that modern women can control their fertility: that we can have careers, delay motherhood, choose when to have babies, or opt out altogether.

Well, it wasn't *just* Sanger: because though she had the vision, she didn't have the money. It was another woman who provided the funding: Katherine Dexter McCormick (1875–1967). While this chapter will go on to tell you about the brilliant men at the scientific heart of oral contraception, it is Sanger with the mission and McCormick with the money who were the mothers of invention. The Pill is their baby.

The story starts in a poor and miserable neighbourhood of New York where Margaret Sanger, née Higgins, was one of eleven children born into an Irish-American family. The endless pregnancies, including seven that ended in miscarriage, combined with poor living conditions and poverty, took a terrible toll on Sanger's mother, who contracted tuberculosis. Sanger left college to nurse her as she was dying, but there was no hope. At the funeral, she confronted her father, a tombstone cutter, across the coffin: 'You caused this,' she told him. 'Mother is dead from having too many children.'

There are more prudent ways of testing your wife's fidelity than by swapping her contraceptive pills with aspirin, but this was the premise for the movie Prudence and the Pill, *which heralded a cultural shift in social mores.*

he

ren.

DEBORAH KERR
DAVID NIVEN
in FIELDER COOK'S
PRUDENCE AND
THE PILL x
A KAHN·HARPER PRODUCTION
COLOUR by De Luxe

H MICHELL · EDITH EVANS
vel. Music Composed and Conducted by BERNARD EBBINGHOUSE

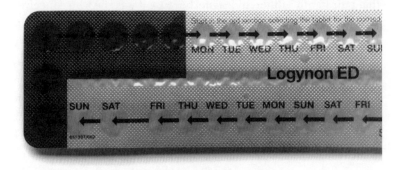

Contraceptive packaging has been steadily simplified, and pill packets are now clearly labelled to help women remember to take it every day.

These early experiences, and the work she went on to do with the poor in the city, left a deep scar. After her marriage to the rich architect Bill Sanger, Margaret started thinking of more political ways of easing the load for women. The contraception that was available was in the hands and power of husbands and male doctors. It seemed to her that the biggest tyranny affecting the lives, health and livelihood of women was that of unplanned pregnancy.

It was Sanger who, in her writings, coined the phrase 'birth control'. Her single-minded pursuit of contraceptive choice saw her reviled, outlawed (to England where she met Marie Stopes – see pages 75–90) and even imprisoned. She sidelined her husband and her three children, one of whom died at the age of six, in order to pursue bigger goals. The opprobrium of society simply provided extra fuel. She published a magazine with the strap-line 'No Gods! No Masters!'

Her tireless campaigning resulted in divorce. But Sanger would later marry the industrialist Noah Slee, who was better attuned to her thinking and whom she persuaded to break the law when he imported the Mensinga Diaphragm (see pages 67–8) through his factories. She even had him illicitly manufacturing contraceptive gels.

And Now the Science Bit...

In the meantime, the United States were moving towards what would be the most extraordinary medical revolution in history, but the pieces were coming together one by one and from different laboratories.

Following the work of zoologist Thomas Hunt Morgan (1866–1945) on the fruit fly, scientists were gaining huge insights into the working of hormones and genes – the science of being a human being. Sanger seized on the information that existed and drove the search for an oral contraceptive.

In 1926, progesterone had been identified by scientists at the University of Rochester as the hormone that prepares the female body for pregnancy. Three years later, at Washington University, Edward Doisy isolated oestrogen as the human sex hormone.

And then, in 1941, the chemist Russell Marker decided to investigate the Mexican Barbasco yam, which was said to have contraceptive properties and had reportedly been used to control fertility since the time of the Aztecs. He travelled to Mexico and spent time with locals finding out how and why they used it. Convinced that the yam must have some hormonal properties, Marker broke it down until he was left with a white powder, which he presented to a pharmaceutical company for testing. Sure enough it was pure progestin, from which progesterone is derived. Marker had put the necessary knowledge in place.

Now all that was needed, as Sanger knew, was a method: someone to work out the correct cocktail of hormones and turn it into a tablet that could manipulate nature's cycles.

The Contribution of McCormick

By this time, Sanger had set up the Planned Parenthood Federation (PPF), which would later become the International Planned Parenthood Federation (IPPF), providing advice on contraception and population control across the globe. It was a lobby, and one that provided a respected springboard.

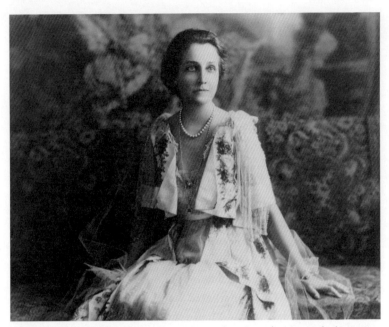

Katherine Dexter McCormick (1875–1967) is the unsung heroine in the history of the contraceptive pill. Her involvement was so little acknowleged that she didn't even receive an obituary.

As she moved into the next stage of her campaign, luck was on Sanger's side. In the most wonderful twist of fate, she received a letter from Katherine Dextor McCormick, one of the first women to graduate from the Massachusetts Institute of Technology.

Sanger knew McCormick as they had met at various events, but they were not particularly pally. McCormick had spent much of her married life worrying that if she conceived, any children might inherit the schizophrenia to which her beloved husband, Stanley, had succumbed two years into their marriage. Stanley was a multi-millionaire, but while he was alive, his wife could not use the money to support those causes that fired her – causes such as birth control.

Following Stanley's death in 1947, Katherine inherited his entire fortune. By 1950, she was sitting on US$15 million and was keen to use it in a positive philanthropic way. She was seventy-five years old.

Indeed, both Sanger and McCormick were well past pensionable age by now, but both were fuelled by a feminist need to improve the lot of their gender. They arranged dinner on Manhattan's Upper East Side, and by the end of the night McCormick had pledged money for research via Sanger's Planned Parenthood Federation – but only if Sanger could find a way of guaranteeing a result in McCormick's lifetime.

Over the next few years, Katherine Dexter McCormick would pour US$2 million – equivalent to more than US$30 million today – into research for a contraceptive pill. The rest, as they say, is history...

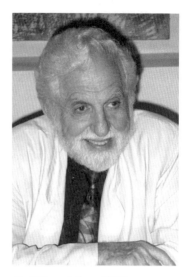

Carl Djerassi (born 1923) was effectively the first chemist to turn synthetic progesterone into tablet form. This was widely presented as a cure for erratic menstruation.

The Breakthrough

Now we come to the fathers of invention. By a quirk of wonderful fortune, even as Sanger and McCormick sat talking over dinner, a brilliant young Austrian chemist called Carl Djerassi was working across the American border in a small Mexican laboratory, perfecting the formula for turning synthetic progesterone from the yam plant into tablets. Unwittingly, and unknown to Sanger, the prototype that still forms the basis of the Pill was in existence.

Meanwhile, Sanger approached the scientist Gregory Pincus in Massachusetts. Pincus, a Russian Jew, was already a leading expert on the mammalian egg and, having been vilified for early work fertilizing rabbit eggs *in vitro*, was glad to meet someone equally absorbed by the secrets of fertility. He listened to Sanger's

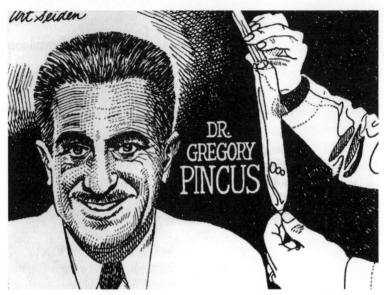

Gregory Pincus (1903–67) had already clearly established the properties of progesterone in regulating rabbit fertility when Margaret Sanger asked him to come up with a contraceptive pill for women.

argument for a birth-control pill, and sagely nodded – he was, he said, sure it could be done.

As often happens, all the strands suddenly started to come together very quickly. With his research partner, M. C. Chang, Pincus started testing progesterone as a contraceptive on rabbits at their research facility, The Worcester Foundation. Within months, he was convinced it worked and he set out to find a tablet form.

The following year, G. D. Searle, an American drug company, announced that one of their scientists, Polish-born Frank Colton (1923–2003), had come up with a progesterone tablet independently of, and differently formulated from, that of Djerassi and Djerassi's backers, Syntex. Both Searle and Syntex now had orally administered synthetic progestin, but still the penny didn't drop… They touted their products as an aid to those with menstruation problems.

Pincus, however, understood the real value. His problem was that he was a scientist, not a physician, and he needed a doctor with a core group of fertile women patients to try out the tablets in parallel with his own work.

Keen to get the idea into the public domain, Pincus approached an obstetrician called John Rock (1890–1984) at a medical conference. He knew Rock was an advocate of birth control because Rock's clinic had breached convention to teach women patients the rhythm method – how to identify the three days during which they are at their most fertile, so they could avoid sex around those times. He went against common ideology but did not break any rules, unlike Sanger, who had endured the opprobium of the world.

Bizarrely, Pincus discovered that Rock was ahead of the game, as he had already been trying out oral progesterone on his patients with huge success. Pincus and Rock agreed to run trials in tandem. Rock ordered Colton's tablets and did one of the biggest practical studies in medical history: documenting it as 'fertility research'. Not one of his guinea pigs became pregnant. By the end there was no doubt: the Pill worked.

But when Rock's trials were published in 1955, nobody picked up on their significance. It was only at the end of that year, when he presented a paper spelling out their meaning to women the world over, that the extraordinary discoveries of Rock and Pincus and all those behind them, were acknowledged.

There were still glitches before the final product went on general sale, and by the time it did, a smidgen of oestrogen had been added to the mix. Ironically, the tablet, the pill known as Enovid, had already been on the market for two years, dispensed in a small brown bottle for regulating periods. It was now approved and repackaged for 'therapeutic purposes'.

The World Gets Ready for the Pill

It's timing was perfect. America was on the cusp of a new age. The 1950s was a period of rapid change. The country was still absorbing the findings of the 1948 Kinsey Reports on human sexuality, which debunked the commonly held view that sex happened mainly

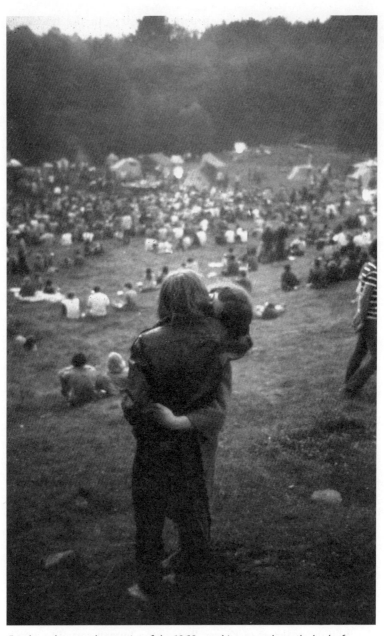

Free love: that was the promise of the 1960s, and it was made on the back of women's sexual emancipation in the wake of the Pill.

between a man and a woman. Kinsey found that it normally happened between an individual and his or her hands... In other words, we pleasured ourselves more than we pleasured, or were pleasured by, others.

This caused people to wonder about sexuality and its meaning, and it spurred the clinicians Masters and Johnson to start researching and preparing their classic study on 'Human Sexual Response', which would argue that it was completely normal for humans to crave and indulge in sexual activity irrespective of their marital status.

But theirs was research. The Pill provided the tool... Indeed, the Free Love movement of the 1960s – Woodstock, the Isle of Wight pop festival, the beat poetry, flower power and general baby-boomer bonhomie – could not have happened the way that it did without the Pill. Would we have had the mini skirt if it wasn't for the confidence that, wherever it might lead, it could only enhance, and not ruin, a woman's life?

The Pill Hits the Streets

The timing was perfect and the pharmaceutical companies were rubbing their hands in glee. We were entering a new cycle of Western culture, thanks to the sheer grit and vision of Sanger, the money and determination of McCormick and the scientific curiosity and vision of those many gifted men in white coats who willingly turned fantasy into reality.

By 1960, the Pill was legal in all but eight American states and the US President, Dwight Eisenhower, declared that '[Contraception] is not a proper political or government activity or function or responsibility.' Searle were cock-a-hoop: it was the green light for a product push. By 1962, 1.2 million women were taking the tablets and the company reported net profits of US$24 million.

Because they owned the formula, they did not have to pay Pincus or Rock a penny in royalties, despite it being their hard work and their research that had opened the door.

Within a couple of years, Syntex too had jumped on the band-wagon using the Djerassi formula. Their product, Ortho Novum, came out in

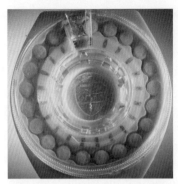

With its round dispenser, the 1960s Ortho Novum pill packet looked like a wrist watch.

1963: the same year that President John F. Kennedy was assassinated. Sanger had threatened to leave the country if Kennedy, a Catholic, did anything to stop the advance of birth control, but he did not.

Ortho Novum was the first pill packet to come in a daily dispenser pack, which allowed women to know automatically whether or not they had taken that day's pill, and when to have the seven-day break. Unlike today's slim foil sheets, the original dispensers were round and clicked each day's tablet into place, a bit like those dispensing machines where you put in the money, punch a code, and the shelves whir round until they find the right product.

By 1965, 6.5 million American women were on the Pill. This is the amazing figure that was imprinted in Margaret Sanger's mind when she died in Tuscon, Arizona, aged eighty-six, the following year.

How the Pill Works

It's a wonderful story. But how exactly does the Pill work?

It's going to sound complicated, but actually we can whittle down the detail to this: there are four lots of hormones that dominate ovulation, menstruation and pregnancy. First there are the two gonadotropin hormones: Follicle Stimulating Hormone (FSH) and Luteinizing Hormone (LH). These are secreted by the pituitary gland and tickle the ovaries into releasing their egg supplies: this is the monthly process we call ovulation.

Nature has built women to reproduce – it's why they're at their sexiest when ovulating. Surveys suggest women even seek out different types of men at that point in the cycle: bigger, butcher, more primal blokes, whom they subconsciously believe will supply rugged alpha-plus babies. FSH and LH are the motivators.

Once the egg is freed, two more hormones take over: progesterone and oestrogen. Oestrogen sets the egg into the womb, preventing early development in the ovary, then it goes back to its desk while progesterone takes over the project management of the pregnancy.

The normal task for progesterone is to thicken the lining of the womb in readiness for the egg to implant. If the egg remains unfertilized, levels of progesterone fall, the lining of the womb thins and is shed in what we call the monthly period.

The Pill uses synthetic hormones to increase progesterone levels, fooling the body into believing ovulation has already taken place. As a result, the gonadotropin glands take time off because it feels like their job for the month is finished. Job done: no egg, no problem.

Because oral contraception stops the body from ovulating, there's actually no physical need for a woman to have a period. You could just take the Pill every day for years and not cause yourself any harm. Yet the accepted form for those taking the Pill is that after twenty-one days of tablets women stop for seven days in order for the womb to discard its lining.

This part of the cycle is as manufactured as the rest: it was built into the process by Pincus. He was keen that the Pill should feel and appear 'natural' to its users. During his trials, Rock had had his volunteers take the Pill every day, which meant no bleeding, but Pincus wanted to reassure women – and the God-fearing authorities – that nature was not being changed, but merely assisted. It is psychologically comforting.

In addition to magically suppressing ovulation, the Pill simultaneously makes a woman's cervical mucus thicker so sperm has to fight harder to get through.

The Pros and Cons of the Pill

Since those early days, the Pill has come out in many different variations, including the Mini-Pill, mixed pills and low-dose pills, to suit the variation in the millions of women in every country on this planet who have come to rely on it. Total figures for the twenty-first

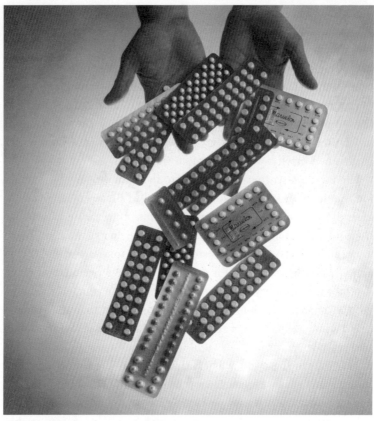

The contraceptive pill is now available in different permutations to suit different needs. For example, older women are advised to use the Mini-Pill, which is better suited to their hormonal balance.

century are inconclusive, but vary from a very low 100 million women to several hundred million worldwide.

Over the last forty years, there have, inevitably, been a number of health scares raised by the constitution of the birth-control pills. As with Hormone Replacement Therapy, there is always a small risk that artificially regulating hormone levels may lead to side effects, including that of turning healthy cells into rogue cells.

The scares have mainly centred on breast cancer and cancers of the cervix, but there are also long-term health gains associated with the Pill. Every woman has to make an informed choice for themself. In general, older women stop taking oral contraception and move to other methods, and for young women the overall risk may seem minuscule compared with the alternatives. If and when the male pill gets the formal go-ahead (see pages 148–51), the prognosis will be even better.

Thankfully, illness and death as a result of child-bearing are no longer part of that list of alternatives. The horror stories commonly heard by the young Margaret Sanger, which inspired her fifty-year crusade, mirrored the plight of her own mother. Sanger's campaining energy had its roots in loss and experience.

Sanger never forgot a young woman she met in her nursing days – a woman who was distraught because she did not want yet another unplanned child. The doctor had told her dismissively to ask her husband to 'sleep on the roof'. Six months later, that same woman died at the hands of a back-street abortionist.

Another woman aged thirty once wrote despairingly to Sanger: 'I've been married fourteen years, and have eleven children, the oldest thirteen and the youngest one year. I have kidney and heart disease and every one of my children is defective and we are very poor... I will surely go insane if I keep this up, but I can't help it and the doctor won't do anything for me.'

Those women and those doctors who did do something will live on in social and scientific memory.

The End of an Era

As the woman who first coined the term 'birth control' and then stamped its meaning and importance onto the world, Margaret Sanger's death in 1966 received huge international attention.

In the space of her lifetime we went from nothing to the Pill. In a poll as we hit the year 2000, Margaret Sanger was listed as the fiftieth most important person in the previous thousand years after leading scientists, such as Newton, Einstein and Galileo, and after major artistic figures, including Mozart and Beethoven. There is no doubt that Sanger's legacy will live on for ever. Gregory Pincus was at number seventy-five.

Gregory Pincus died shortly after Sanger in August 1967. He contracted myeloid metaplasia, a disease of the white blood cells, from laboratory chemicals. He was sixty-four.

Four months later, Katherine McCormick died quietly in Boston, aged ninety-two. Her death did not merit a single line in the press, but John Rock's wife said of the redoubtable financier: 'She carried herself like a ramrod. Little old woman she was not. She was a grenadier.'

John Rock lived to the ripe old age of ninety-four, dying in 1984 at his home in Temple, New Hampshire, leaving behind five children and fourteen grandchildren. Although he was delighted that he had saved further generations of women from suffering the prolapsed wombs, worn bodies and poverty of his earlier patients, he was despondent that his once beloved Catholic Church continued to oppose dedicated contraception. During his lifetime, Rock did much to try and influence Papal thinking, but eventually lost his faith because of doctrinal rigidity. Today, the Catholic Church officially retains the same position.

Frank B. Colton, the man who created the Pill, died in quiet retirement, aged eighty, in 2003. Whereas Carl Djerassi, aged eighty-one in 2004, continues to be excited and exalted by a new world where every medical dream is within the bounds of possibility. And, as women opt for other synthetic progestin-based alternatives – be it the Mirena Coil (see page 57) or under-skin implants (see pages 154–55) – his name, too, remains set in stone.

Abortion
Shutting the Door after the Horse has Bolted

The Last Resort

Welcome to the most controversial section of this book – not because of the information contained therein, but because the subject matter inevitably leads to passionate and angry debate. We have entered the dark space known as abortion.

Abortion is not a new concept, as this chapter shows. And, in many ways, it is preferable to the cruel resolutions opted for in ancient cultures where there was no recourse to medical help if a woman found herself unhappily with child.

In more recent history where rudimentary help was available, women risked their lives to seek illicit release from the burden of yet more unplanned children. At one point, more women died through illegal abortion than childbirth.

Equally terrible are stories of women who want their unplanned children, but have them forcibly expunged. There are stories from modern China, where laws have been introduced governing family size, of women having full-term babies forcibly aborted just days before the due date.

In England, abortion can be broken down into two different categories. The first is emergency contraception, which comes in the form of direct action in the days immediately after unprotected sex has taken place. The speed with which emergency contraception is administered means that the woman seeking help has no idea whether or not her actions might result in a pregnancy, but does not wish to take the risk.

The second is termination, which is the removal of a fetus from the womb where an unwanted pregnancy has been confirmed.

It is not an easy decision or procedure at any level.

The Arrival of the Soul

No method of contraception is totally fail-safe, so there is always scope for an accident –from burst condoms to forgetting a pill; from sickness diminishing the effectiveness of oral contraception to a failed withdrawal. There's also the possibility of a miscalculation when using the rhythm method; and then there's the most likely reason of all: a total inability to heed the need for contraception in the heat of a sexual moment. Shit happens, as they say. What then?

It's at this point that we move into the most controversial area of contraception – abortion and its derivatives, which include drugs, such as the morning-after pill, that prevent an egg from getting a toe-hold in the womb lining *after* intercourse, rather than before.

Abortion is a difficult topic because it excites such furious argument. Because the pro-life movement is so closely allied to the Christian religion, it's easy to assume that those who uphold abortion as a sin are perpetuating beliefs that go back thousands of years. In fact, the pro-life debate is far more recent and relates to arguments of ensoulment: that is, the point at which an embryo ceases to be a mass of cells awaiting determination, and becomes essentially human – the moment the cells absorb a 'soul'.

Muslim scholars have suggested the soul enters the child's body at around four months. Islam does not condemn abortion in the first 120 days after conception, although some breakaway groups disagree. Muslim women were, historically, allowed contraception, and abortifacients were used with impunity.

The big debate about ensoulment has its roots in the thinking of the Catholic Church. In the fifth century, St Augustine engaged in a dialogue in which it was clear he believed that the fetus was part of the mother's body and did not have a sentient identity of its own. His arguments were so unpopular within the faith that, later, in a bid to discredit this view, a faked Augustinian statement was circulated suggesting that attempts to discourage pregnancy were a form of homicide. However, in the sixteenth century, when Pope Gregory XIII was in charge, the Catholic Church upheld the Augustinian view.

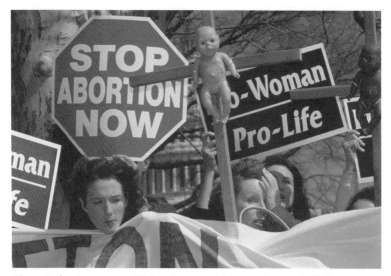

The anti-abortion movement is largely supported by creationists who believe that an egg has a 'soul' from the moment of fertilization. Pro-life groups have emerged across the Western world to campaign for an end to abortion on demand.

Gregory's guidance was that an embryo was not human before ensoulment.

Things changed when Gregory was succeeded by Sixtus V, who declared all abortion to be murder. In other words, ensoulment takes place as soon as the sperm has fertilized the egg, and any dissolution is effectively homicide. In doing so, Sixtus V declared war on the perceived paganism of the local midwives and brought women under the control of the Church.

In 1869, Pope Pius IX reiterated the words of Sixtus V. Four years later, the Comstock Laws were introduced in America (see pages 69–71).

Abandoned Babies

In the ancient world, littered though it was with philosophers and great thinkers, there were no such ideas or illusions. Even the new-born child had no rights if its family could not afford it, or if it showed signs of some disablement that devalued its contribution to the general good.

Roman law defined the unborn child as *spes animates* – a being with aspirations to ensoulment – but that only happened once the baby arrived in the world. In ancient Rome, men who impregnated concubines and slaves allegedly threw them down stairs to induce abortion. Even when it came to their legitimate families, the decision whether or not to keep an unplanned or initially unwanted child was made at the point of birth – the baby was laid down and only if the father lifted it up was it welcomed into the family.

Otherwise, the child was left outside the home for others to either adopt or enslave. Ironically, a quarter of the babies that were kept died in their first year, and only half lived beyond the age of ten.

In the absence of birth control, some Aboriginal and Native American Indian tribes left newborn babies to die because their untimely arrival impeded mobility in the wild. In Athens and Sparta, handicapped babies were left out for the wolves. The same was true in Ancient Rome. One has only to look at their statuary to see how they idealized the human form.

Even in these supposedly civilized times, not much has changed. Although we no longer kill handicapped children, the disabled were sent to concentration camps as part of Hitler's programme of ethnic and social cleansing in the 1930s and 1940s. From Romania in the early 1990s came heart-rending film footage of physically or mentally defective children thrown into orphanage cots and left there in a state of living atrophy.

Terrible stories have emerged about the so-called 'Dying Rooms' in China where newborn baby girls, abandoned by women under pressure to produce boys, were brought up in a state of terrible neglect. Under Chinese law, each couple is allowed only one child, and has to apply for a licence to conceive. Baby girls, referred to as 'maggots in the rice' because they leave home on marriage and don't repay the cost of their upbringing, are unwanted. Abandoned babies taken to State-run orphanages were tied to beds before they could even walk. One child allegedly had her hand chewed off by rats.

But leaving children to be found is not the same as infanticide, and infanticide is not the same as abortion. This is mentioned merely to show how civilizations that did not have recourse to contraception or abortion dealt with unwanted children, whatever the reason for their births.

The Right to Abort

In Christian Germany and France, the issues around abortion fuelled angry debate in the late 19th and early 20th centuries. As in Britain and America, the movement for women's rights was part of a feminist push for women to be accepted as equals, and the arguments for birth control and abortion on demand ran in parallel with the demand for women's suffrage.

Those arguments were propelled in Germany by Helene Stocker and Marie Stritt, and in France by militant campaigner Madeleine Pelletier (1874–1939) at a time when, paradoxically, the Industrial Revolution had changed and strengthened the role of women within society, but had also put them under pressure to increase the birth rate and push up the number of bodies working in the factories.

It was not until the 1960s, however, that the female voice was strong enough, and the

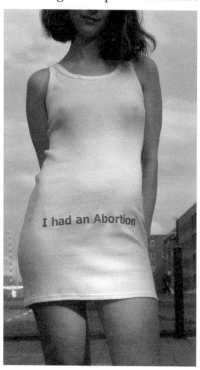

The stigma of abortion in England was removed to some extent by the 1967 Abortion Act, which made termination of a fetus under twelve weeks medically and socially acceptable.

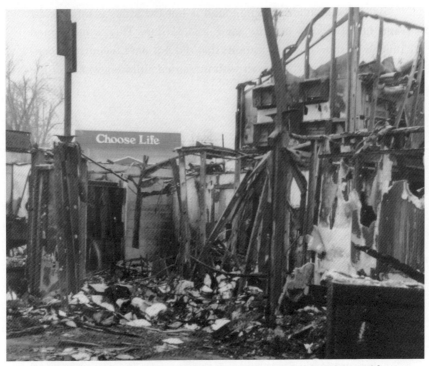

In the United States, the debate over abortion has become so bitter that pro-lifers take extreme action against those who facilitate abortion, often through arson attacks on abortion clinics, as occurred here in Kalamazoo, South Michigan, to promote the pro-life argument against abortion law.

male psyche attuned enough, for abortion to be legalized. Part of the incentive was provided by the Thalidomide cases. Thalidomide was a drug prescribed for women suffering from debilitating morning sickness. It resulted in scores of babies emerging from the womb with terrible limb deformities, and was subsequently banned.

There is no suggestion that those babies should have been aborted, but it highlighted the issues around pregnancy and rights over what happens in and to one's body. Added to the huge women's lobby demanding abortion rights, the Thalidomide furore provided the extra fuel necessary for the British Liberal Party leader at the time, David Steel, to push through a law in 1967 that made abortion legal in special cases in the United Kingdom. In America, similar changes were taking place.

And yet, even though we effectively have abortion on demand in the twenty-first century, we have created a climate where it is easier to admit to having the clap than to having had a pregnancy terminated.

From the beginning of the 1970s, protest groups started questioning the wisdom of the law. In Britain this took the form of debate and the development of an articulate and passionate pro-life lobby, which continues to argue for the rights of the unborn child. In America, it took the form of a violence that steadily escalated.

In the 1990s there were several murders and numerous attempted murders outside American abortion clinics. There were over 105 bombing and arson attempts. Protestors regularly hurled abuse at staff and patients and threatened them with violence and death. If we take 1997 as an example, there were nearly 8,000 incidents of picketing outside American abortion clinics, and over 2,000 bomb threats and hoaxes. All this was despite a law introduced specifically to deter protestors by giving courts the power to levy fines of up to US$100,000 and one-year prison sentences.

That opposition to abortion continues, despite the endless horror stories that predate Abortion Acts in both countries. It's worth remembering that there was a point in the nineteenth century when more women died from botched abortions than in childbirth.

DIY Abortion

But, without recourse to contraception, the vacancies remained for back-street abortionists. Who can forget Denholm Elliott as the grisly back-street abortionist in the 1960s film, *Alfie*?

Compared to some of the options on offer, the back-street abortionist, shown at his most humane and humorous through the ether-sniffing John Irving character Wilbur Larch in his novel *Ciderhouse Rules*, was positively benign. And yet a huge number were charlatans. In 1936, the Abortion Law Reform Association was set up with the express intention of reducing the number of deaths through illegal abortion.

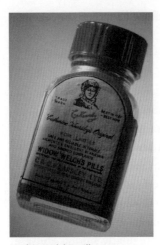

Widow Welch's pills were a concoction that relied mainly on Epsom salts for efficacy.

There are many old wives' tales of do-it-yourself abortion: the insertion of knitting needles or drinking neat gin while sitting in a hot bath being two examples. In the east, some cultures used the stem of *ricinus communis*, the castor oil plant, which is long, strong and flexible, to irritate the opening of the cervix until the womb expelled any embedded fetus.

Then there are the ideas that follow from lateral thinking – women deliberately doing heavy and frenzied exercise in the hope of shaking the embryo loose. Among the more bizarre ideas utilized by our forebears were the drinking of Epsom salts, the swallowing of quinine water in which a rusty nail had been soaked and ingestion of the foam from a camel's mouth.

The midwives of old, many of whom got burnt as witches in a series of changes that saw men taking back control of women's bodies, used abortifacient plants, such as marjoram and lavender, parsley and thyme. These were brewed up in strong concentrates and imbibed by those wanting to dislodge fetuses.

The song lyrics, 'Are you going to Scarborough Fair, parsley, sage, rosemary and thyme' are a veiled reference to herbal contraception. And Scarborough Fair is, according to research, a euphemism for shagging, screwing, bonking, getting rogered, making out and all the other euphemisms that we use for 'sex'.

Pennyroyal tea, mixed with blue cohosh (a plant native to America), was a well-known emmenagogue – that is, effectively, a morning-after recipe for preventing the embryo from rooting in the uterus. Emmenagogues bring on menstruation – thus forcing the womb to shed its lining and dislodge any foreign bodies (or natural bodies) therein.

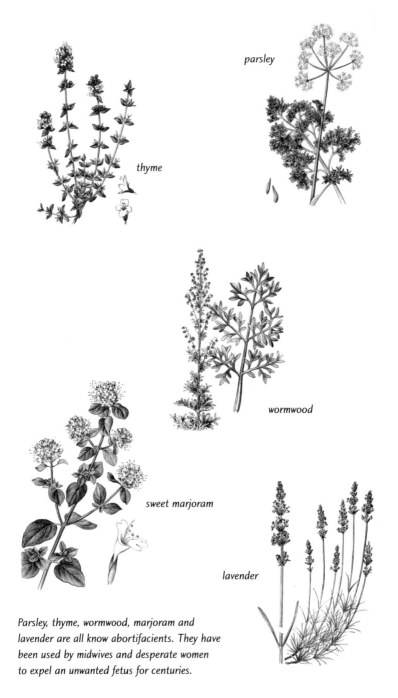

parsley

thyme

wormwood

sweet marjoram

lavender

Parsley, thyme, wormwood, marjoram and lavender are all know abortifacients. They have been used by midwives and desperate women to expel an unwanted fetus for centuries.

In 1995, a young American student died after allegedly trying a do-it-yourself abortion using Pennyroyal tea. The stomach cramps she experienced masked the symptoms of a fatal ectopic pregnancy. The lyric from the song *Pennyroyal Tea* by rock-band Nirvana is also alluded to on page 27.

Other emmenagogues include potions using manganese, tansy, juniper, rue, thuja oil, iron, quinine, strychnine and boric acid. Mustard poultices applied to the pelvic region (ouch!) apparently have some effect, as does the ingestion of Spanish fly, otherwise known as the beetle *cantharis vesicatoria*.

Wormwood was a favourite remedy in Europe and was also used by the ancient Greeks. The French called it the 'prostitute root', presumably because ladies of the night were regular users. It is also known as green ginger and absinthium, and is an ingredient in absinthe, an alcohol that can cause severe hallucinations. Indeed, it has been suggested that the painter Vincent Van Gogh (1853–1890) committed suicide while under its influence.

Professional and Medical Abortions

All of these and many more remedies have been around for hundreds, if not thousands, of years. In the lava-covered remains of Pompeii, dilators and curettages going back 2,000 years have

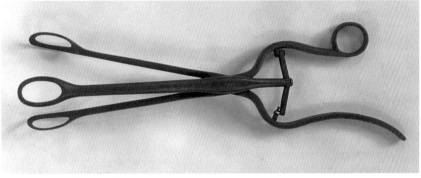

The standard tools for scraping the womb are still a dilator and a curette. This old-fashioned dilator would have been used to gain access to the womb.

The seaweed laminaria, known as seatangle, was used to induce abortion by inserting the plant into the neck of the womb where it would expand to four times its size, thus helping to expel an unwanted fetus.

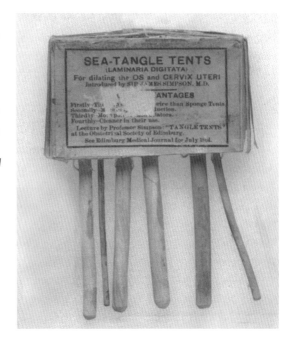

been found, suggesting a level of sophistication in its termination industry.

Dilators and curettes (hence the term 'having a D&C') remain the instruments of termination even in modern times, but these simple tools are only safe in the hands of the medically qualified. The numerous women who were permanently damaged or even died at the hands of a back-street abortionist – many of them not even medically qualified – are a testament to the skill involved.

Nowadays, all abortions in the United Kingdom are carried out under proper medical conditions, either within the NHS or by private clinics. But it was not until 1967 that women in Britain were given the legal right to have an abortion. Although technically available on demand, it remains a complex process requiring the approval of two doctors before it is deemed in the woman's interest not to go ahead with a pregnancy.

Even then, abortion is only available in the first trimester: that is, in the first twelve weeks of pregnancy. Generally, an anaesthetic is administered, and the woman is given a D&C where the lining of her womb – the endometrium – is scraped and the implanted embryo dislodged and removed. The after-effects include discomfort and some bleeding.

It has been suggested, however, that more than one abortion can sometimes affect future fertility and, as with any invasive procedure, there is a small risk of infection. All women who ask for abortions are counselled about their decision and what is involved, as some women suffer from depression or regret after terminations.

At around twelve weeks, the fetus starts having brain waves. After that point, abortion is available only for medical reasons. Those reasons increase in gravity the closer a fetus gets to the upper abortion limit of twenty-four weeks. At this stage the issues are not to do with failed contraception, but the baby's health or that of the mother.

In other cultures, concern has been voiced that women are having late abortions because the child is the wrong sex – specifically, because the child is a girl and may cost a family in terms of dowry or later earning ability. The procedure beyond sixteen weeks is extremely distressing, with women having to undergo a forced labour to expel the fetus.

The Morning-after Remedies

Since the invention of the morning-after pill, however, those women who have knowingly had unprotected sex have a fall-back. And since 2001 women can nip along to the local chemist or to the pharmacy counter at their local supermarket and buy a packet of RU44, commonly known as the morning-after pill or emergency contraception. Before 2001, these pills had to be prescribed, warranting a visit to a doctor or family-planning clinic.

Emergency contraception is effectively a concentrated dose of the contraceptive pill. It pumps the woman full of hormones, mainly progesterone, thus changing the chemical balance of the womb so that the egg is disabled from implanting itself and fertilizing.

For this reason, it must be taken, at the very latest, within seventy-two hours of intercourse. If an egg has already embedded, the

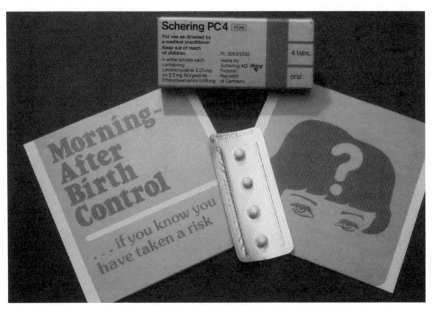

The controversial morning-after pill is now available over the counter in the United Kingdom. The pill contains a massive dose of progesterone, which makes the womb lining inhospitable to any egg.

morning-after pill does not dislodge it. Conversely, as the majority of women who buy the morning-after pill will not be pregnant as a result of their single mistake, it is as much a comforter as a contraceptive.

For those who are put off at the thought of refined chemicals pumping through their bodies, there is a natural pessary on the market called XPL7, which claims to work on exactly the same principle. XPL7 is inserted into the vagina using a plastic applicator (as is normal with anti-fungal pessaries), and is made up of safe, edible plants. Up to four are inserted over a period of time.

There are no studies to say whether or not XPL7 works, but natural remedies, as we know, can and do work. Indeed, the synthetic progesterone we get in the Pill and morning-after pill comes from the Mexican yam that was used as a contraceptive in Aztec times.

A lot of people get emergency contraception confused with RU486, which works as an abortifacient. RU486 is one of the new generation

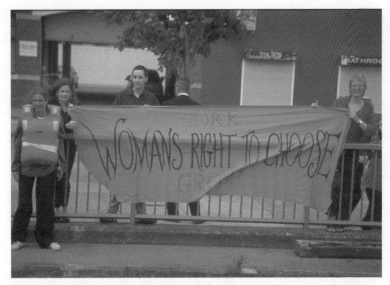

Irish women welcome the Dutch medics with the organization Women on Waves, who sailed to Dublin in 2001 to offer the 'abortion pill' to women with unwanted pregnancies, thus striking a blow against Ireland's restrictive abortion laws.

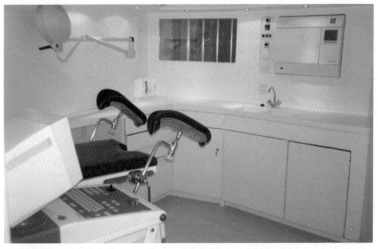

The floating surgery of the Women on Waves boat, where women can be examined, advised and helped without leaving the country. Thousands of Irish women flock to Britain to receive abortions each year.

of anti-progestins. An anti-progestin is a drug that works against (*anti*) the progesterone in a woman's body. Progesterone (*pro* – in favour of; *gestare* – to carry) is vital for conception. Unlike the Pill, which increases progesterone levels and tricks the body into thinking it has just ovulated, RU486 works by blocking all the progesterone that's there, thus fooling the body into thinking the monthly cycle is over. As a result, the progesterone in the endometrium thins, and the lining of the womb is shed, taking the implanted embryo with it.

Although RU486 can be taken up to nine weeks into a pregnancy, the procedure isn't as simple as it looks. Popping pills means women can bypass a surgical procedure, but the tablet has to be followed up with a dose of prostaglandin, which speeds the process, and a level of observation by a doctor is required over two days. Shutting the door after the horse has bolted is never going to be an easy option.

Abortion Laws

Abortion is still not an option to many women in the Western world. Canada has banned the abortion pill and in the whole of Ireland (Northern Ireland and Eire) all abortion is outlawed.

In the 1960s the Maeve Binchy novel *Light a Penny Candle*, which told the tale of an Irish girl who came to London to terminate a pregnancy, was a bestseller. In 1992, an Irish fourteen-year-old rape victim who was suicidal because her attacker had impregnated her, had to take her case to the Supreme Court before she could get leave to fly to England and have a termination. A few years later, the same thing happened with a thirteen-year-old.

Abortion has become such an issue in Ireland – even birth control is frowned upon – that in 2001, a boat full of Dutch medics sailed into Dublin. Manned by the non-profit organization Women on Waves, the ship's doctors offered terminations using RU486 to any woman who wanted it. They claimed that Irish law breaches the human rights of Irish women. That same year, over 6,000 Irish women, the majority aged between 20 and 34, travelled to England to have legal abortions.

Even where it is legal, abortion is made deliberately difficult so that younger women do not see it as an alternative to taking precautions and it remains the option of last resort. The morning-after pill, however, fits in differently to the picture as a whole and has been embraced as a fall-back option for those who, for whatever reason, did not organize effective contraception at the time of intercourse. However, the morning-after pill remains prohibitively expensive, and involves answering a series of personal questions, often in the middle of a crowded shop.

The debates of history continue meanwhile, with opposers in the United States still maintaining physical campaigns. In the United Kingdom the Abortion Law Reform Association is still active, arguing that women themselves should be the only ones to make a decision about abortion and that it is not a freedom if two doctors have to rubber stamp every termination.

Abortion is a contentious area, depending on belief systems and personal anxieties, but it does prevent thousands of unwanted pregnancies every year across the Western world. The opposition's argument is that there are two bodies to be considered: the one that will form in the mother's body, as well as that of the mother herself. It will forever be, one suspects, an unresolved issue within the area of birth control.

Whither Contraception?
Looking to the Future

Let Me Count the Ways...

What's so interesting when considering the long-term prognosis for birth control is that it is probably not going to change very much. In the last 3,000 years, the options on offer have remained broadly the same. The only difference is that medical knowledge and the development of a range of birth-control methods means that today there are enough back-ups built in to ensure it will work.

The historical path to modern birth control is a long one. To begin with, the Sumerians in Mesopotamia, the crucible of civilization, handed out the joy plant – opium – along their trading routes, which came to be used as a barrier method by some of those peoples to whom it had been gifted.

Along the way we've passed the Egyptians, who impressed us with their grasp of physiology, and the ancient Indians and Chinese, who followed in their wake.

From the time of the ancient Greeks and Romans, lifestyle choices, including birth control, are easier to trace. In the Christian era and thereafter there are moral frameworks implicit in the use and construction of birth-control methodology across Western cultures. Yet alongside this were other belief systems and hidden tribal peoples, each finding enlightenment in their own way.

This chapter necessarily concentrates more on men – because that's where we have failed to make significant advances. Genetic fingerprinting and the decline of welfare hand-outs have resulted in larger numbers of men being forced to accept social and economic responsibility for their part in making babies – planned or otherwise. In the past, birth control may have mattered less to them for physiological and social reasons, but it matters now.

The good news is that there are many hopeful leads. The bad news is that none have quite made it to the finish line. But hope springs eternal.

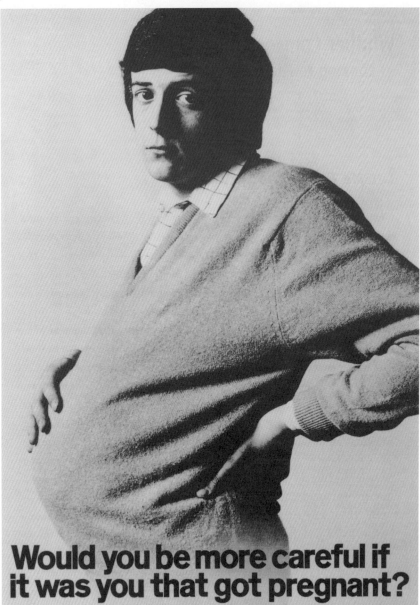

Would you be more careful if it was you that got pregnant?

Anyone married or single can get advice on contraception from the Family Planning Association. Margaret Pyke House, 27-35 Mortimer Street, London W1 N 8BQ. Tel. 01-636 9135.

The Health Education Council

Contraception in the Developing World

It may seem out of place in what is ostensibly a history of contraception to take a look forward, but given the nature of our peregrinations – and having spent several chapters considering ways of destabilizing the motility of sperm and the rolling out of eggs – it's fun to engage a crystal ball and look ahead instead of back.

Funnily enough, real crystal balls made from rose quartz do actually represent both male and female: the cloudy parts of the crystal are the female ying, and the clear parts, the male yang. They do not, however, have any bearing on birth-control methodology beyond advising you whether it's best to save your Agent Provocateur smalls for someone who's tall, dark and handsome or small, blond and verging on average.

What is obvious is that yesterday is already history. When you wake up tomorrow, today will have been added to its pages. On that basis, the implants, implements and procedures of the future do have a bearing on a retrospective, because each day brings new advances.

But it's easy to forget that the majority of women and men in this world still do not have the knowledge or access to the birth control they need, often because it is too expensive, banned by their governments or considered morally undesirable, and so is excluded by taboo. Part of the way forward, then, is to continue to meet these challenges.

One journalist emerging from a newly liberated Afghanistan spoke of how an excited woman there had asked her to confirm that, in the West, there was a pill that could stop women from having babies.

Of Afghan origin herself, the reporter looked around and realized how terrible it would be to confirm that a contraceptive pill existed when she was with a group of women with dozens of loved but unplanned children who, for economic, political and cultural reasons,

This celebrated Family Planning Association advert designed by Saatchi and Saatchi in the late 1970s attempted to bring responsibility for fertility back into the male domain. It hasn't yet worked with those British males who were targeted, but increased fears about child maintenance costs may now swing the balance.

were unlikely to ever have access to self-administered birth control. 'I told the woman no such pill existed,' she admitted afterwards.

In Afghanistan, 1,700 of every 100,000 women who give birth die in labour. That compares with nine per 100,000 in the United Kingdom. Sixteen thousand Afghan women die each year from pregnancy-related causes. One of the major triggers is serial conception in circumstances unsuited to such physical rigours.

Ideological Barriers to Western Aid

But the hurdles to such enlightenment still remain, even in the Western world. After the inauguration of George W. Bush in 1999, Margaret Sanger's prized organization, the International Planned Parenthood Federation (see pages 115–16), had to close down birth-control clinics in impoverished countries because of a law known as GGR: the Global Gag Rule.

GGR prevents American organizations working abroad from using their funds for abortion-related activities. As a result, all overseas birth-control centres came under a shadow: emergency contraception, however rarely used, is part of a smorgasbord of choices offered to those who come to IPPF clinics in the bush or rural townships for help.

When the IPPF celebrated its fiftieth birthday in 2002, it was with a vociferous and continuing campaign against GGR. The crusading legacy of its founder continues to fuel today's work. It is a reminder to those of us who have never questioned our rights as women – as human beings – to control our bodies, that we should never take those rights for granted.

In Britain, the debate that kicked off in the twenty-first century was that on the British law that denies abortion on demand to women living in Northern Ireland.

Unlike Eire, where the powerful Roman Catholic Church still influences policy, including that of outlawing abortion, Northern Ireland is part of the United Kingdom and has a mixed religious heritage. Margaret Pyke's Family Planning Association emerged into a new millennium demanding that women of the province should have the same rights as their sisters on the British mainland.

Marie Stopes International (MSI) is involved in global campaigning, and in England it is the largest provider of birth-control care outside the National Health Service. In 2002, nearly two years after United Nations forces entered Kabul, MSI opened Afghanistan's first dedicated Reproductive Health and Safe Motherhood clinic. Perhaps the Afghan woman who approached the journalist with such excitement will have now discovered that the Pill really does exist. Hopefully, she and others like her will also have discovered methods such as the IUD that are far more helpful for those living in rural areas where women cannot easily visit clinics on a regular basis to top up medical supplies.

And that's what we're researching now in terms of future contraception – methods that not only build on what we have, honing ever more sophisticated mixtures and implements, but new methods that can cater for different lifestyles, belief systems and wallets.

Sterilization and Ovulation Kits

Sterilization, for example, is already carried out in minimally obtrusive ways. The problem is that successful reversals of the procedure in both men and women are rare. On that basis, sterilization is an option only for those who already have children, or those who have clear medical, social or philosophical reasons for a route of last resort.

Given that infertility *is* the only guaranteed means of total birth control, scientists are looking at ways that the process could be reversed without lasting damage. Inevitably there will be a point where a young man or woman can just have the natural processes switched off until they're ready to go for the permanent option.

Another system that will ultimately be reversed to help with birth control is the ovulation kit. Ovulation kits are currently used to let women know when they are at their most fertile. They are effectively versions of the rhythm method reduced to Ph sticks that predict when a woman is about to ovulate.

The sticks detect a surge in Luteinizing Hormone (LH) (see page 123), which indicates that the best window for attempting conception is in the following thirty-six hours.

Technically, the procedure should also be able to tell you when not to make love. But because each woman is different, their surge patterns may vary, or their eggs may stay in the womb for a few hours longer than normal. On that basis, while it's safe to say 'Yes, you can make love like rabbits', it's completely unsafe to say 'As you're having an LH surge now, you'll be able to have unprotected sex with impunity after the thirty-six-hour fertility window.' Such claims would leave manufacturers open to lawsuits from customers whose cycles were different from the norm.

Once we have data that is accurate for each individual, however, it will be possible for any woman to know when she is at high risk of pregnancy so that all artificial contraception, apart from willpower, can be ditched.

But why is it always women? For so long there has been talk about a male Pill. Every couple of years there'll be a moment when someone claims they're close and it will get a few headlines and a mention on the news – and then it fizzles away to nought.

The Hormonal Male Pill

To be frank, the introduction of a male Pill will probably make little difference to women, and market research shows that women do not trust men to take any contraception that requires daily forethought. But for those men who are both responsible and keen to avoid an appointment at the Family Court, it would be a godsend.

The most obvious solution is to trick the male body into switching off sperm production in the same way that the Pill tricks a female body into holding back its eggs. Initially, researchers gave men all manner of testosterone pills, which should, in theory, have sent a message to the gonads that sperm stocks were full and caused the production machinery to stop. They didn't work.

Scientists then isolated a hormone called prolactin. 'Lact', of course, comes from *lac*, the Latin word for milk, hence lactation meaning the secretion of milk in the breasts during pregnancy and after childbirth. Men don't make milk, although their bodies contain prolactin. However, some newborn baby boys may leak milk from their nipples, just as some newborn girls leak menstrual blood.

The idea followed through by scientists was that if they could inhibit the production of prolactin in men, while also playing around with testosterone levels, they would reach a point of critical hormonal mass where it all came together and resulted in the testicles producing, well, nothing. That didn't work either.

Recent efforts involving the use of two hormones, testosterone and the progestin desogestrel, which is also used in the female contraceptive pill. Other hormones used in the mixes are etonogestrel and levonorgestrel. This effectively mimics the technology at play in the female Pill and there have been heartening successes.

At the end of 2003, the ANZAC Research Institute declared that tests of a male contraceptive on fifty-five couples had resulted in a 100 per cent success rate. Australian doctors injected men with the progestin DMPA which cuts testosterone production, thus rendering sperm infertile. There was only one problem: men need testosterone for their sex drives...

To get round this, volunteers were also given testosterone implants that replaced part of what was taken away. In this way, volunteers still experienced desire, but with curbed fertility. At the end of a year's trial, not one had got his partner pregnant.

This is a huge advance in the area of birth control, and the first Western solution that has been workable. However, there will have to be bigger samples tests and a refining of the product before it can come on the market: firstly because the two factors have to be combined and turned into either pill form or injection, and secondly because manufacturers are not convinced that there is big enough demand for a male pill or derivative thereof...

Market research has shown that women don't feel that they can rely on men to take contraception that requires prior planning, and the big pharmaceutical companies are of the same mind. The only takers, it is assumed, will be those men already in steady and responsible relationships where the woman is currently the one using a hormonal contraceptive. Is that enough of an incentive to spend millions, or even billions, on larger scale research and development?

The Herbal Male Pill

The Chinese and the Brazilians have got a little closer in their search for a male Pill. Scientists in both countries have extracted pigment from the root and stem of the cotton plant and issued it in tablet form. The yellow pigment, Gossypol, is also known as cottonseed oil and is a natural toxin that prevents insect attack. It has traditionally been used as an herbal abortifacient for women, but it also destabilizes the lining of the testicles, thus disrupting and stopping sperm production.

In the 1970s, after centuries of anecdotal evidence that families who cooked with cottonseed oil suffered fertility problems, the Chinese Government decided to have Gossypol tried out as a male contraceptive. Government researchers began a major study, but it soon became clear that large numbers of men who took the drug successfully did not regain full sperm production when they came off the course.

In addition, there were all manner of debilitating side effects: renal malfunction, fatigue and even paralysis. These problems could be alleviated by giving the men high doses of potassium, but the risks far outweighed the result and by the late 1980s the Chinese Government had abandoned the idea. On the basis of these findings, the World Health Organization called for all Gossypol testing to stop.

This didn't stop the Brazilians from having a go with a much lower dosage tablet. In 2000, they reported excellent results. Research studies showed that taking oral Gossypol could prevent all sperm production within sixteen weeks of a man starting the course. And, in general, the male body returned to normal levels of production within a year of stopping. But that was only in general. A number were still infertile twelve months on.

So it's only workable in its current form if you aren't bothered about children either way, although Gossypol clearly has benign potential. It is used in all manner of medication, including cancer drugs and the treatment of endometriosis in women. Whatever the World Health Organization rulings, it will almost certainly continue to be used in increasingly refined research.

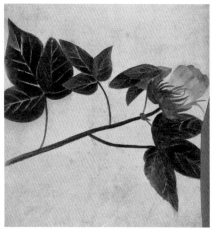

The cotton plant is the source of Gossypol, a natural toxin that has produced extraordinary results in localized testing, striking all users infertile. Unfortunately, it causes a number of unpleasant side effects that makes its use inadvisable.

Vasectomies and Plugs

But not all research with men relies on hormonal solutions. In the 1970s, work was done to see if sperm could be halted in its tracks or siphoned off by the insertion of magnetic metal valves into the *vas deferens* – the tubes where sperm is made and stored. It sounds like an extremely painful procedure, and the results were not sufficiently good to bring in funding for further research.

But the Chinese, while failing with Gossypol, have been much more successful with permanent solutions. They have perfected the no-scalpel vasectomy, whereby men can be sterilized under local anaesthetic using only forceps and a haemostat. They are also able to give men percutaneous injections, which involves clamping the *vas deferens* and injecting it with sclerosing chemicals that block the tubes, thus preventing sperm from getting through.

For those men who don't seek permanent infertility, the Chinese also boast a 'plug' method, whereby a polyurethane gel is injected into the *vas deferens*. This method comes under the umbrella heading RISUG, which stands for Reversible Inhibition of Sperm Under Guidance. Once the gel sets it acts as a plug, stopping sperm from getting through the *vas deferens* and into the penis. When the men are ready to have children, the plug is flushed out and everything returns to normal. This method can only be repeated once, but has proved successful.

However, injecting a plug requires skill and careful training. As there are millions of men in China for whom this is a dream option, the effort involved by their medical professionals is worthwhile. It has yet to take off in the West, though. New trials are currently under way in India.

More recently, a new form of RISUG called 'the shug' has been tested and is being touted as the ultimate alternative to vasectomy. In tests it has been 100 per cent effective. Working on the same principle as the plug, it effectively has two checkpoints instead of one, guaranteeing no leakage at all, and can be removed if required.

Microchips and Hot Water

Moving the debate on only slightly, a future possibility must surely be that men could be fitted with transmitters that would regulate the level of activity in the testes, thus doing away with procedures that require invasive procedures involving the *vas deferens*. Similarly, women could be fitted with microchips that send signals to the ovaries sanctioning egg release only if and when the woman wants to try for a child.

We know already that microchips can be used to send signals to the brain, and are being tried out to help replace and regenerate damaged nerves; there is talk of regenerating those who have suffered paralysis in this way. Is it any more outlandish to imagine that we could use it to govern other functions?

All of these have got to be better than the solution offered by a Dr M. Voegeli who, in 1946, suggested that men should soak their bollocks in hot water for forty-five minutes a day. At the end of three weeks, the doctor said, a man would be sterile for six months.

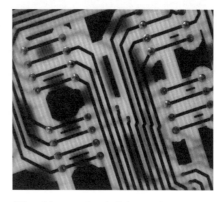

Although this sounds crazy, there is method in the madness: heat *does* kill sperm. It's one of the reasons men are told not to wear underpants that hold their testes too tightly: tight pants can cut sperm production down by seventy-five per cent. Conversely, common advice to men with infertility problems is that they soak their testes in icy water each day to improve motility of sperm.

Microchips are already being used experimentally in the regeneration of nerve tissue, and ultimately they should be able to govern other bodily functions, such as sperm release.

Let's face it, though: the idea of spending large periods of the day sitting on a pot of hot water is not one that's ever going to take off.

The Sugar Pill

An ingenious idea currently being tried by an American doctor is the Sugar Pill. When sperm binds to an egg, it does so because it recognizes a special sugar enzyme in the egg's outer coating. Once they're bound together that's it – you can't separate them after collision – fertilization occurs.

The Sugar Pill mimics the woman's body sugar. The man takes the pill and his sperm immediately attaches to the absorbed sugar before leaving for the woman's body. The sugar is harmless to the man, and in animal trials has proved ninety-eight per cent successful. Research continues.

The biggest problem when trying to find a solution that involves males is that so little of available funding is spent on male oriented contraception – less than 10 per cent. That said, the future must surely hold better ideas…

Implants

Implants are already available to women and have also been tested for men. The main problem with implants is psychological: while they remove the anxiety of having to take a daily hormonal cocktail, they require the permanent presence of a foreign body in the human body. It's one of the problems encountered with women and IUDs, and there's nothing to suggest that men would be any more receptive.

There have been workable implants on the market for women for the last two decades. Female progesterone implants are placed under the skin of the upper arm. They come in the form of six small rods containing capsules of progesterone, which is released on a microscopic and continuous basis for five years. Despite their low take-up, implants have proved to be highly successful in preventing pregnancy, and they are effective almost immediately.

But, as is the norm with most hormonal contraceptive remedies, there is a risk of symptoms, such as irregular periods, weight gain, hair loss or more intense period pains. Interestingly, men trying out hormonal solutions have also reported weight gain and lower HDL (a benign cholesterol) levels.

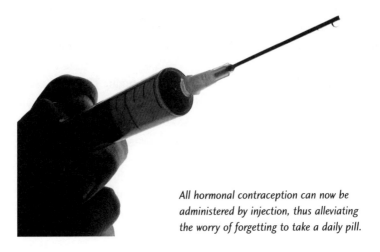

All hormonal contraception can now be administered by injection, thus alleviating the worry of forgetting to take a daily pill.

Another remedy tried out on men and available to women is a hormonal patch that works on the same principle as the Pill. The problem is that users must be highly organized and reliable as the patch must be changed weekly and, like the Pill, includes a week off.

Those women who don't mind returning to the doctor or a clinic on a regular basis can, of course, get hormonal injections in the form of Depo-Provera and Noristerat. Both are forms of progesterone, the former requiring a quarterly top-up and the latter every six weeks. Side effects are the same as those when starting the Pill – irregular bleeding and occasional spotting. Again, as advances are made, methods of injecting for longer-term effectiveness will be found, and that may act as an incentive to get more women considering injection as a viable option.

Sci-fi Solutions

There are also sci-fi type ideas that will sound outlandish at this moment in time, but not necessarily so in another twenty years...

American researchers have already successfully recreated a human womb in a laboratory. Statute forbids scientists from growing external embryos beyond two weeks (indeed, in 2001 President Bush introduced laws that prevent virtually all embryonic research in government-funded facilities), but embryos placed inside the reconstruction of the womb showed all signs of bedding down and preparing to grow normally.

What is the likelihood that in fifty or a hundred years' time, women will opt to have their wombs removed and when they're ready to have children, their fertilized eggs will be grown externally in their own womb? As surgeons have already perfected a technique for performing a hysterectomy (the removal of the womb and Fallopian tubes) through the navel, by laparoscopy, the procedures involved will not necessarily be onerous.

The other option is that they will simply have a new womb generated from their own cells when they are ready for a child. This would make women both infertile and fertile simultaneously.

This has eerie shades of Aldous Huxley's novel *Brave New World*, where all children are grown externally on laboratory production lines, graded for the type of worker they will be, but gene science moves us towards such possibilities every day. What's scary about more recent movies, such as *Gattaca* and *Minority Report*, is that we know much of the technology already exists (iris scanners, DNA testing for disease, mapping of genetic characteristics), and that which doesn't exist is being developed.

Earlier in this book we had a jolly canter through the properties of amulets and how they were used as magic props to ward off the evils of pregnancy. In the future, who's to say we won't be wearing amulets that emit high-frequency radio waves that discourage eggs from releasing or sperm from multiplying?

Meanwhile, focusing on the next ten years for ease of purpose, the Pill, the darling of hormone-changing contraception, continues to be refined and re-formed in new and different ways. We already have the morning-after pill; it wouldn't take much, one would think, to come up with a minute-before-pill that does exactly the same thing without the associated abortifacient issues that surround the use of any emergency contraception.

Emergency contraception (see pages 138–41) is now more acceptable, despite the opposition. RU486, or Mifepristone, which is currently used as an abortion pill, has been shown to be an effective morning-after pill too – except it can be taken up to five mornings after the dreaded and unprotected deed, and users will not risk the nausea currently associated with the RU44, or Levonelle, which is available over the counter.

Condoms may come in paint-on versions that feel like you're going bareback, and caps will no doubt be worked on so they can be kept inserted for several days without discomfort or mess. Currently, researchers are testing condoms in new materials that may have an even longer shelf-life than latex.

And so it goes on... The more we understand about the human body, the better able we are to reverse, divert, mimic and refashion its natural functions. The history of contraception is also the future of contraception, and the issues and ideals that have fired each step forward will continue to be argued over by our children and our children's children – all of whom, one hopes, are planned and wanted, and will have had their contraception choices laid out to them before entering the fray of coupling and copulation.

Sources and Resources

I am indebted to a number of extraordinary books by learned writers whose diligence provides the bedrock of modern birth-control knowledge. I have also gained some of my education on the internet through some excellent websites devoted to birth control and the issues that surround it.

Books

Bernard Asbell *The Pill: A Biography of the Drug that Changed the World*, Random House (1995)

Emma Dickens *Immaculate Contraception*, Robson Books (2000)

Angus McLaren *Twentieth-Century Sex: A History*, Blackwell Publishers (1999)

John M. Riddle *Eve's Herbs*, Harvard University Press (1977)

G. L. Simons *The Illustrated Book of Sex Records*, Putnam Publishing Group (1983)

Websites

American Botanical Council, Burkhard Bilger:
www.herbalgram.org

American Experience/The Pill: www.pbs.org/wgbh/amex/pill/

Brook: www.brook.org.uk

Durex: www.durex.com

Family Planning Association: www.fpa.org.uk

Frontiers in Non-Hormonal Male Contraception, Elaine A. Lissner:
www.gumption.org/mcip/paper.html

The Hall of Contraception: http://desires.com/1.6/Sex/Museum/museum1.html

Inconceivable Practices, R. I. Chalmers: www.thewordmaster.co.uk/Mayfairarticle.htm

International Planned Parenthood Federation: www.ippf.org

Lesley Hall's Condom Page: http://homepages.primex.co.uk/lesleyah/condoms.htm

Male Contraceptives.Org: www.malecontraceptives.org/index.htm

Marie Stopes International: www.mariestopes.org.uk

Medicine/Smith Papyrus/Ebers Papyrus: www.crystalinks.com/
egyptmedicine.html

No Gods! No Masters! Doris Dwyer: ww.wncc.edu/~dbaldwin/
history/chautauqua/nomasters_dwyer.html

Spartacus Educational: www.spartacus.schoolnet.co.uk/women.htm/

World Sex Records: www.world-sex-records.com

Yale-New Haven Teachers Institute, essay by Kathleen London:
www.yale.edu/ynhti/curriculum/units/1982/6/82.06.03.x.html

Picture Acknowledgements

Corbis: 129

David Cottridge: 41

Carl Djerassi: 117

Illustrated London News: 82, 85

International Information Centre
and Archives for the Women's
Movement: 14, 67 (both)

Margaret Pyke Memorial Trust, 14, 88

Marie Stopes International: 14, 66,
75, 79, 80, 96, 100, 101, 109, 114,
124

Alan Marshall: 106, 107

Mary Evans Picture Library: 12, 22,
28, 30, 37, 44, 60, 77, 81, 84,

Museum of Contraception,
Toronto: 9, 21, 47, 48, 49, 53, 56,
63, 71, 92, 99, 137

Museum of Menstruation and
Women's Health (www. mum.org):

64, 65

Planned Parenthood Federation of
America, Inc.: 11, 14, 14, 69, 70,
116, 132

Powerhouse Museum, Sydney,
Australia: 26, 31, 33, 43, 122, 134

Redferns Music Picture Library: 120

Saatchi & Saatchi: 144

Art Seiden: 118 (From *Jewish Heroes
and Heroines of America*, by
Seymour Brody)

SSL International: 16, 103, 104

David Tipling: 41

Twentieth-Century Fox/BFI: 112

Wellcome Trust: 20, 23, 35, 39, 73,
94, 97, 136, 139, 151

Women on Waves: 131 (Willem
Velthoven), 140

Index